# The Art of Xingyiquan

## Li Jianqiu

The Art of Xingyiquan

Copyright © 2023 by Chen Faxing, translator

English translation copyright © 2023 by Chen Faxing

All rights reserved. No part of this book may be reproduced or transmitted in any form or by any means, electronic or mechanical, including photocopying, recording or by any information storage and retrieval system, without permission in writing from the publisher.

Published Independently.

ISBN 9798391584926

Printed in U.S.A.

First Edition

Cover design by Chen Faxing

Disclaimer for Martial Arts:

The practice of martial arts, including Xingyiquan, involves physical activity that may carry risks of injury or harm. Readers are advised to consult with a physician before beginning any martial arts training, especially if they have any pre-existing medical conditions or injuries. The authors and publisher of this book disclaim any liability for any injury or damage that may result from the use or application of the techniques and principles described herein.

Disclaimer for Exercise:

The exercises and practices described in this book are intended for educational and informational purposes only. They are not a substitute for professional medical advice, diagnosis, or treatment. Readers should always consult with a physician or qualified healthcare provider before beginning any new exercise program or modifying their current routine. The authors and publisher of this book disclaim any liability for any injury or damage that may result from the use or application of the exercises and practices described herein.

# The Inaugural Declaration of the Basic Principles of Xingyi Quan

The most unfortunate and painful thing in life is to have a weak body and a depressed spirit. The happiest thing is to have a healthy body. There are two ways to achieve a healthy body: through exercise and through spiritual cultivation, such as the practice of seated meditation. Various forms of exercise equipment and Chinese martial arts such as staff, sword, stone locks, and double-weighted barbells belong to the category of exercise. However, both methods have their drawbacks. Sitting meditation can lead to mental illness due to excessive contemplation, while excessive exercise can lead to a decrease in intelligence. This is due to a lack of understanding of the principles of physical education. In recent times, both Eastern and Western civilizations have emphasized physical education as a science. Sports scientists advocate for the simultaneous training of the body and mind to achieve a balanced development of one's physical and mental capacities, which can enhance one's personality. The newly created flexible gymnastics is based on these principles, but its theory of physical education is sound while its techniques are not yet perfect. Friends advised me to study martial arts, and soon I felt a transformation in my physical and mental well-being. Chinese martial arts can simultaneously cultivate both the spirit and body, which conforms to the principles of physical education. However, many who are interested in martial arts lack education, and intellectuals are not willing to learn. In the fifth year of the Republic of China, Wu Zhiqing and I founded a martial arts club, inviting like-minded individuals to join us in studying and practicing martial arts. Our reputation grew, and we were eventually invited by the National Education Conference to integrate martial arts into the regular curriculum of our schools and establish vocational schools to train warriors. At first, our club was located in a rented house with few members, but today we have thousands of members and our own building. We train daily and send our teachers to teach in primary and secondary schools, even to elderly women with bound feet. This shows that martial arts have many benefits and no drawbacks when practiced in schools, especially in promoting physical health. From the beginning of our club, we recognized the advantages of Xingyi Boxing, which was not promoted in the South. We wrote to Master Chen Zizheng of the Tianjin Boxing School, and he kindly introduced us to two teachers, Liu Qixiang and Chen Jing'e, who were then working in the Commercial Press Club and had founded a national martial arts research club. Dozens of people joined our morning exercises, and fortunately, we have had no negative effects over the past five years. However, our efforts have been inadequate, and we are ashamed of this. Now we and our fellow club members have vowed to strengthen ourselves, our fellow countrymen, and our nation. As the saying goes, "If you want to maintain your natural simplicity and a dispassionate attitude in life, you should not seek fame, wealth, power, or the right to live and kill arbitrarily. Instead, you should be benevolent to others, and the world will be benevolent to you."

- Shanghai National Martial Arts Research Association: Li Jianqiu, Huang Fanggang, Wu Zhiqing, Huang Jinggu jointly declare on behalf of all members.

The oldest Chinese martial art is passed down from a time when culture was valued over martial arts, but scholars did not give it much attention, resulting in practitioners being mostly uneducated and unable to fully develop the art. In recent decades, due to promotion in schools, there has been a revival of interest in Chinese martial arts. However, some practitioners focus solely on the form and not on the spirit, leading to a lack of practicality. The Xing Yi Quan style emphasizes the union of form and spirit, and is said to have been created by Yue Fei. It focuses on practicality and does not prioritize aesthetics. Although it is initially easy to learn, it is difficult to master, and can improve health and longevity. Li Jianqiu and Huang Fanggang are experts in this art, and have compiled this book based on their experiences teaching it at Tsinghua University. Huang asked for a foreword from me, even though I am not an expert in this field.

-   In November of the eighth year of the Republic of China, Jiang Weiqiao delivered a speech at the Yiyuan in Beijing.

# <u>Second Preface to The Art of Xingyiquan</u>

The strength and weakness of the physical constitution of the people is related to the prosperity and decline of the country. Westerners regard sports as one of the three major elements. The Chinese people also pursue this. Therefore, the whole country emphasizes sports, and there are no weak ones. Since ancient times, our country has admired literary style and neglected military preparations. Martial arts have long been abandoned and unused, resulting in a weakening of the people's physical fitness. Those who ponder on this lament it greatly. Wang Junjun, Zhang Junyuanzhai, and Li Junjianqi are all giants in Xingyi, and they are concerned about the decline of national culture and the lack of vitality in sports. They have long thought about advocating Xingyi martial arts. Now, Li Jun will use the secrets he has learned through decades of experience to study carefully, compile them into a book, and promote the development of martial arts, making it popular throughout the country. This will help cultivate the people's courage and physical strength, eliminate the decadent trend of weakness in literature, and enable us to compete with the great powers. As soldiers, we often engage in close combat. The weak are often stabbed by the strong, even if it takes a long time, the strong can endure and eventually win. This is a clear proof of the importance of physical strength. Today, Mr. Jianqiu has worked hard to rescue the weak, and his merit is truly immeasurable. He has entrusted me to write this preface. After reading the book, I found the language to be precise and the words to be insightful. I was even inspired to dance with my sword. It is truly a masterpiece in the field of sports literature in recent times. Therefore, I pick up my brush to write this preface.

- At the beginning of winter in the year of Siwei, Bao, Yang, Li, Haiquan wrote a preface together with Zhang Xueyan from Anping.

## Author's Preface

Xingyi Quan originated from Bodhidharma in the Northern Wei Dynasty and was passed down to Yue Fei, the military strategist of the Song Dynasty. He often combined spear and fist techniques to teach his generals, naming the style Xingyi. The name Xingyi has been used through the Jin, Yuan, and Ming Dynasties, but the history of its transmission is unclear. In the late Ming and early Qing Dynasties, Ji Gongji, also known as Longfeng, sought out a master on Zhongnan Mountain and obtained the Quanpu (fist manual) of Yue Fei from the martial strategist Wu Muwang. He then taught it to Cao Jiwu, who in turn taught it to Ji Shouxian. Ji Shouxian wrote a preface for the martial strategist Wu Mu's Quanpu and spread it to the world, which is the Xingyi Quanpu used today. At the same time, Ma Xueli in Luoyang also obtained the transmission. During the Xianfeng reign of the Qing Dynasty, Dai Longbang and his younger brother Lingbang both learned the art from Ma Xueli's family and mastered the technique, becoming famous in the Shanxi area. In the late Qing Dynasty, Li Luoneng, after nine years of studying Xingyi Quan with Dai Longbang, traveled back to his hometown and taught his students. Many people followed him, and Xingyi Quan in Zhili Province originated from Li Luoneng. After Li Luoneng's death, his successors included Liu Qilan, Guo Yunshen, Che Yonghong, Song Shirong, Bai Xiyuan, and others who had mastered the essence of Xingyi. Liu Qilan passed it down to his three sons Jintang, Dianchen, and Rongtang, as well as his disciples Li Cunyi, Zhou Mingtai, Zhang Zhankui, Zhao Zhenbiao, Geng Jishan, and others. Guo Yunshen passed it down to Liu Yongqi, Li Kuiyuan, and others. Li Cunyi passed it down to Shang Yunxiang, Hao Enguang, his son Bintang, and others. Zhang Zhankui passed it down to Han Muxia, Wang Junchen, Liu Jinqing, Liu Chaohai, Li Cunfu, and his son Yuanzhai. Li Kuiyuan passed it down to Sun Lutang, Yu Shuzhu, and others, including my ancestors Wenbao and Yunshan, who both studied under Li Cunyi and Zhou Mingtai. I learned Xingyi Quan from my family because I was often sick as a child and traditional medicine did not work for me. Xingyi Quan not only cured my illnesses but also improved my health significantly. The usefulness of Xingyi Quan is beyond doubt. In the first year of the Republic of China, Liu Dianchen, Li Cunyi, Zhang Zhankui, Han Muxia, Wang Junchen, and others founded the Wushi Hui in Tianjin and promoted the study of martial arts in Beijing. Later, Sun Lutang also made significant contributions to the development of Xingyi Quan. However, I believe that the spread of this art has been limited to the northern regions, and even Sun's book has not been widely circulated. Despite my limited knowledge, I still decided to write this book.

- On December 19th, 1919, Li Jianqiu wrote this preface in Shulu.

In the teaching of Western learning, there are moral education, intellectual education, and physical education. The purpose of physical education is to train the spirit of martial arts to strengthen the body, which in turn strengthens moral character and enhances intelligence. Therefore, physical education is sufficient to lead both moral and intellectual education. This is why Sparta places such great emphasis on physical education. Children as young as seven years old enter the sports field to practice high jump, running, wrestling, javelin throwing, and ring throwing. Their customs value martial arts, and their people are brave. By following their system, China can be saved from its accumulated weakness today. However, this cannot be accomplished easily. There must be a true transmission of ancient methods and excellent guidance from experienced teachers. Only then can one achieve an indestructible body like a diamond. Although these teachings have been transmitted to the West, their methods are actually similar to those of the Northern Wei Dynasty. This is because Bodhidharma, the ancestor of the Shaolin Temple, had this technique, which was passed down to Song Yue, King Mu of Wu. He transformed the technique by combining boxing and spear techniques and named it "Xing Yi Quan". Although Xing Yi Quan has been passed down through generations, its writings are not widely known. Only Mr. Sun Lutang has written about Xing Yi Quan. Mr. Li Jianqiu from Shulu is also proficient in this technique and has been teaching it at Tsinghua University for many years. After seeing Mr. Sun's work and admiring his knowledge, he was afraid that his teachings would not be widespread, so he wrote this book based on his experience. It is a true transmission of Bodhidharma and King Mu's technique, and it is still relevant today. It is indeed a valuable resource for future generations.

- In the summer of the year Gengshen (1920), the man from Bailongshan, Wang Zhen, wrote this preface.

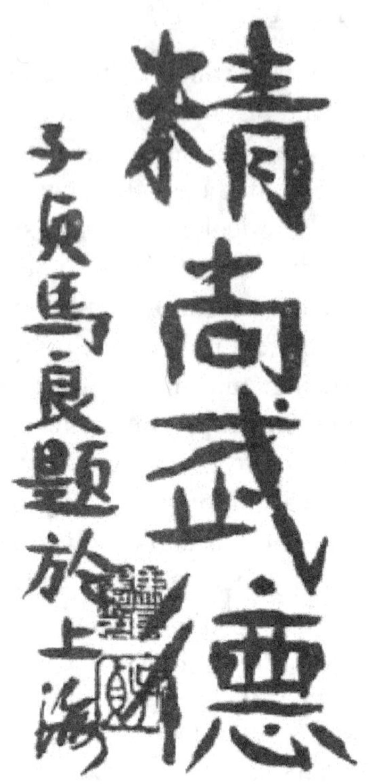

*Dedication to martial arts and virtue.*

Ma Liang inscribed this at Shanghai.

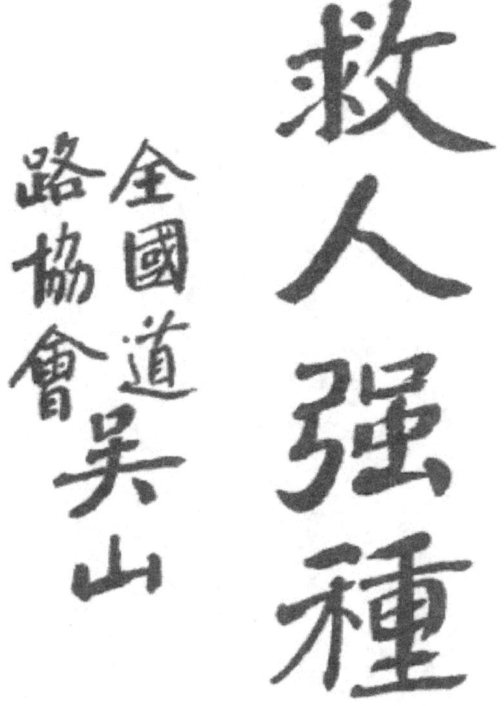

*Saving people and strengthening the race.*

National Road Association, Wu Shan.

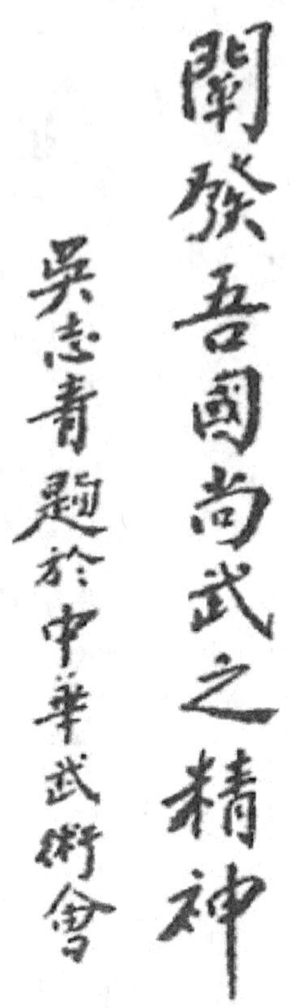

*Developing the Spirit of Martial Arts in Our Country*

Wu Zhiqing's inscription at the Chinese Martial Arts Association.

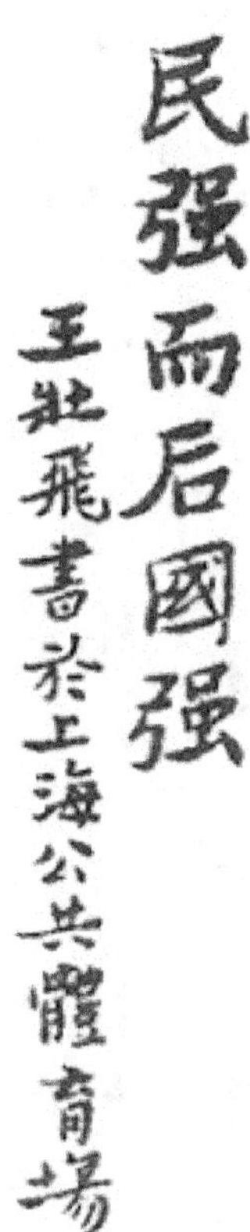

*The people must be strong before the country can be strong.*

Wang Zhuangfei wrote at the Shanghai Public Sports Field.

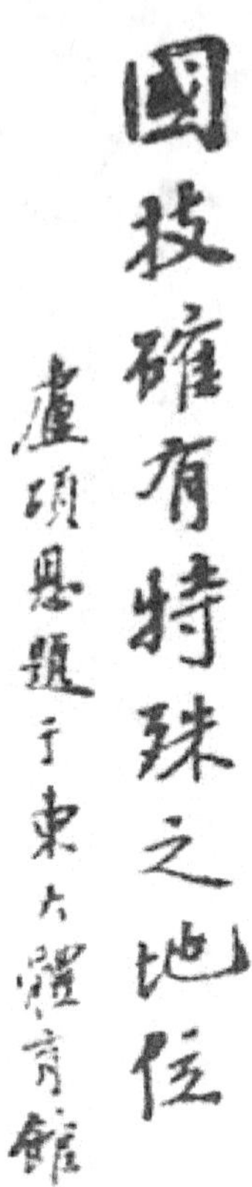

*National martial arts have a special position.*

Lu Shuo's inscription at the East University Gymnasium.

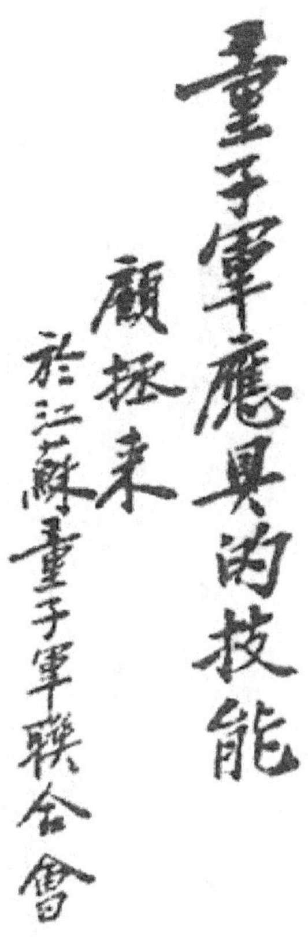

*Skills that Boy Scouts should possess.*

Gu Zheng, Jiangsu Boy Scouts Association.

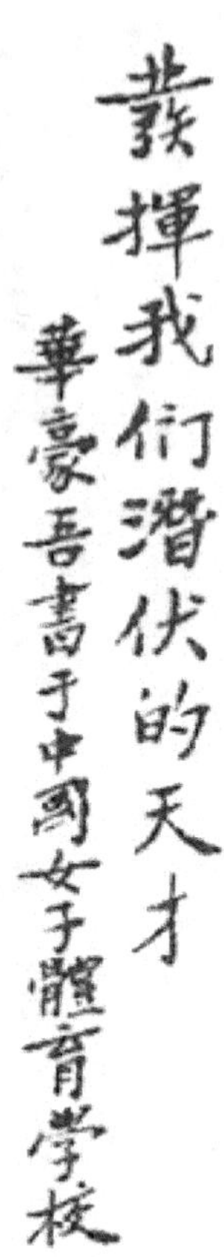


*Unleash our hidden talents.*

Hua Hao wrote this at the Chinese Women's Sports School.

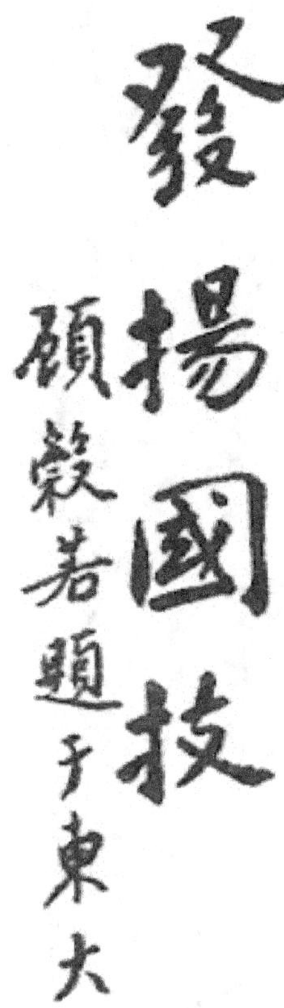

*Promote national sports.*

Shuo Guoruo wrote this in Dongda.

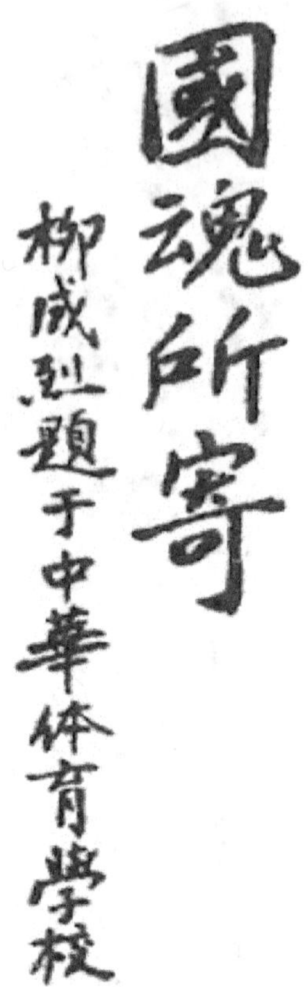



*The soul of the nation rests here.*

Liu Chenglie's inscription at the Chinese Sports School.

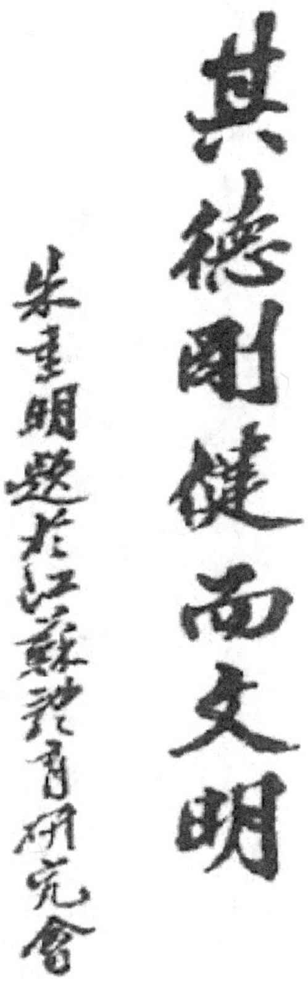


*Its virtue is strong and vigorous yet civilized.*

Zhū Chóngmíng's inscription at the Jiangsu Sports Research Association.

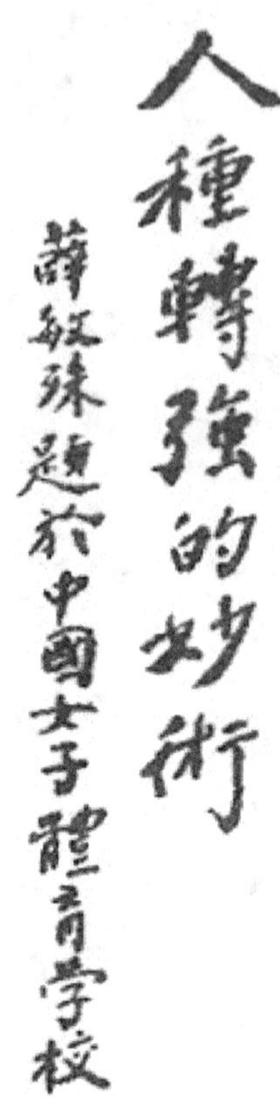



*The art of strengthening the race.*

Xue Minshu's inscription at the Chinese Women's Sports School.

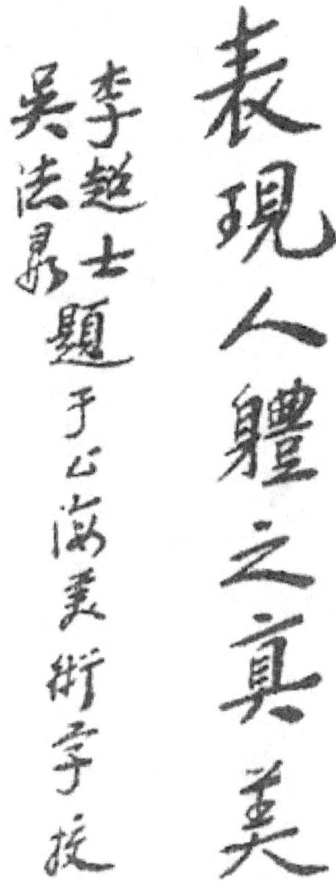



*The true beauty of the human body on display.*

Li Chaoshi and Wu Fading inscribed at the Shanghai Academy of Fine Arts.

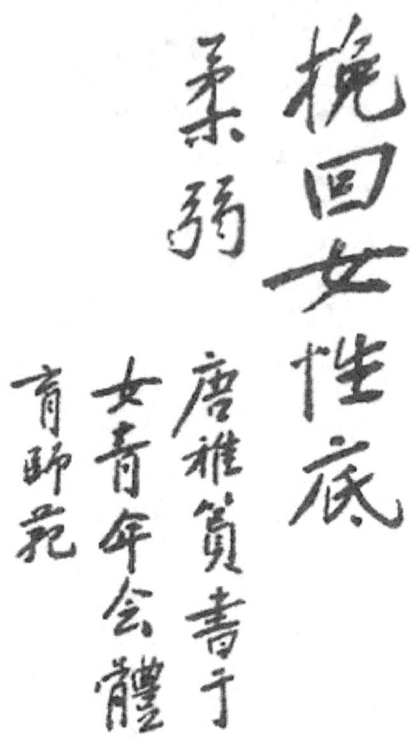



*Rescue the inherent weakness of women.*

Ms. Tang Zhihui wrote at the Women's Youth Association Physical Education Normal School.

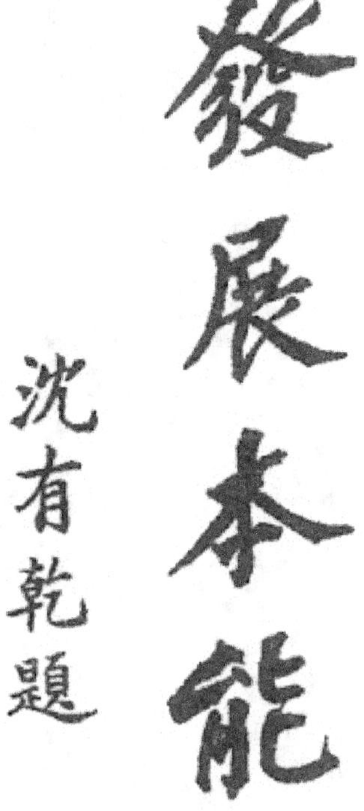

*Develop instinct.*

Shen Youqian's inscription

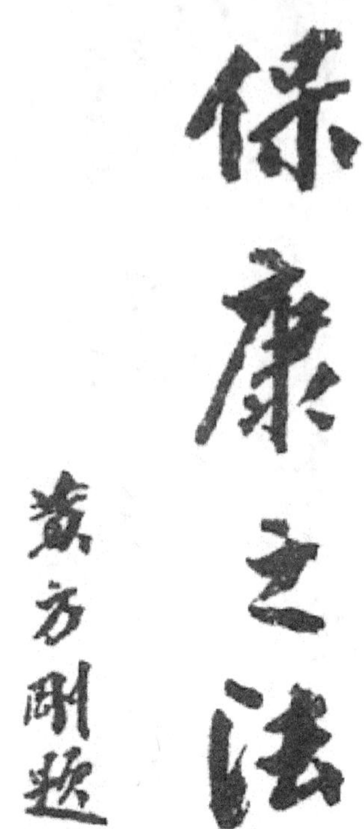


*The method of protecting health.*

Huang Fanggang's inscription

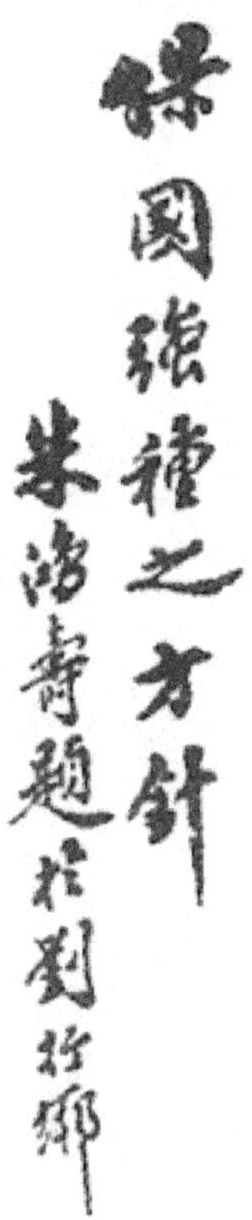

*The policy of strengthening the country through strong descendants.*

Written by Zhu Hongshou in Liu Xingxiang.

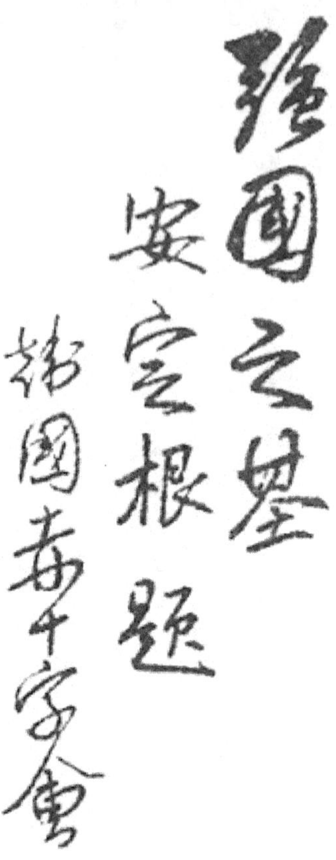


*The foundation of a strong country.*

Stele Inscription by An Dinggen for the Korean Red Cross Society

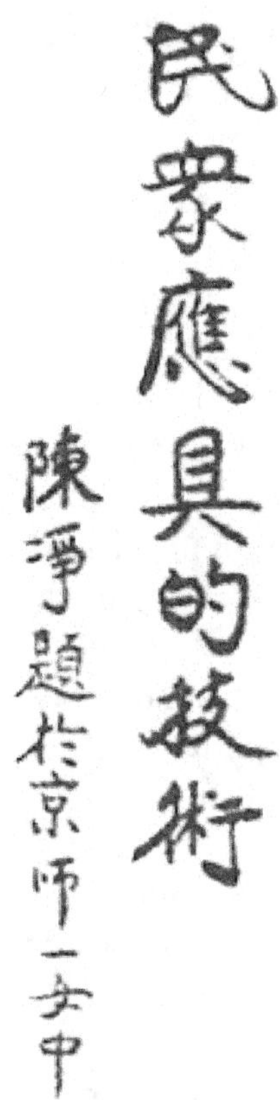

*The techniques the people should possess.*

Chen Jing inscribed on Beijing Women's Middle School.

<u>**Preliminary Rules of Xingyi Quan Technique**</u>

1. Xingyi Quan has five element fists, twelve animal forms, and various routines such as the linking fist and mixed style pounding fist, as well as paired routines such as the five element overcoming fist and anchoring cannon. The five element fist is the foundation of all Xingyi Quan, and the other forms are derived from it. The late Guo Yunshen was a Xingyi expert and skilled in using Beng Quan to attack opponents. He believed that the reason why ordinary boxing is inferior to Xingyi Quan is that it is flashy but not practical. However, in the process of creation, it can still be used. It is just that it eventually becomes complicated and loses its original intent. Therefore, it is feared that Xingyi Quan will follow this trend of becoming too fancy and lose its essence. It is important for learners to focus on the basics and develop their own techniques. This is why this book provides an introduction to the five element fist and the linking fist, and the purpose of including the linking fist is to provide learners with the opportunity to practice combining five different routines in their spare time. This shows the variation of boxing techniques. As for paired routines, since there are no fixed rules for sparring and it is difficult to describe them in writing, learners can practice and discover various techniques with partners after having a basic understanding of the five element fist. There is no need to rely solely on books.

2. In the Five Elements Boxing, each boxing has a consistent principle but different postures. Different postures make it easier to learn, but consistent principles make it harder. When beginners focus on one type of boxing for a year or half a year, they will have a better understanding of it. Then, when they start to learn other types, it only takes a few days to learn the postures because the consistent principles have already been understood. Therefore, even though it takes only a few days to learn the postures of other types, it is not inferior to the one-year or half-year training of one type. The reason is that the difficulty in learning is not in the postures but in the understanding of the principles. Once you understand the principles of one type, you can easily understand the principles of other types. Therefore, just focus on learning the postures of other types and make them consistent with the principles you already understand. This approach is more efficient,

and beginners should start with the Splitting Fist, as it is the basic posture for every boxing. Without learning Splitting Fist, you cannot learn other types of boxing.

3. Three, before the main discussion in this chapter, a few words are written as an introduction, which is the general summary and the first two chapters.

4. In this sixth chapter of this book on Xing Yi Quan, the key points and its research are discussed. Only one or two examples are given for study, while many others are not written down. It is hoped that students can carefully study and scientifically research them one by one.

5. Attached are important discussions and sparring techniques in the Xingyi Boxing Chart, which contains many essential phrases and some difficult-to-understand words and sentences due to the changes over time. Students must carefully examine them.

# Table of Contents for The Art of Xingyi Quan

<u>**General Introduction**</u>

The use of martial arts is great - to strengthen the body, defend against external threats - this is the essence of it. It is truly the quintessence of our country, but very few of our people can actually practice it. In the past, scholars were focused on studying for the imperial exams to obtain official positions, while craftsmen and merchants lacked knowledge and learning. Therefore, few people paid attention to the practice of martial arts. Even if it is passed down, it is difficult to popularize. Outsiders even mock and ridicule us for it. In the face of the rise of modern weapons, martial arts has become even less important. However, foreigners living in our country are amazed by our martial arts and some even learn and bring it back to their own countries to show their people. It is said that this is due to the curiosity of ordinary people. However, the value of martial arts cannot be denied, and this alone is evidence of its worth. If our people want to determine its value, they need to know what to choose and what to study. Only then can they obtain it.

# Chapter 1: The Function of Martial Arts

Long-distance running, short-distance running, long jump, high jump, hurdles, pole vault, shot put, discus throw, javelin throw, soccer, basketball, tennis, swimming, parallel bars, pommel horse, and various other sports all have areas of strength that are biased. For example, in running and jumping, the lower body exerts more force than the upper body, while in shot put and discus throw, the arms and shoulders exert more force than the legs and feet. If one practices these sports, the development of muscles and the increase of energy will be limited to certain areas, while other parts that have not been trained will not benefit. Moreover, if one wishes to practice all of these sports to gain all the benefits, it will take up a lot of time and require a well-equipped facility. However, if one practices boxing, the whole body is used, and the mind is focused, the body is agile, the neck is flexible, the abdomen is solid, and the spirit is united. With determination and perseverance, one can benefit greatly from practicing boxing. Boxing can not only protect oneself but also protect others, uphold justice, and promote chivalry. The benefits of practicing boxing are not only special but also more advantageous than practicing other sports.

<u>**Chapter 2: The Function of Xingyi Quan**</u>

The function of martial arts has been discussed in the previous chapter, and the function of Xingyi martial arts is no different. Xingyi martial arts are not only superior in practical application to ordinary martial arts but are also easy to learn for men, women, and children as long as they have the will to do so. How do we know this? Because there is no leaping or rolling around, just a focus on practical use, and not on impressive moves. This shows that it is not difficult to learn. If one can achieve mastery, even those stronger than oneself can be easily defeated from a distance, controlling the enemy with ease. The effectiveness of Xingyi is not only limited to this, but it can also make the mind sharp and agile, which can prevent illness and extend life, and also enable one to achieve success in the world. This is the greatest function of Xingyi martial arts.

<u>**Chapter 3: The Five Basic Forms of Xingyi Quan**</u>

The Five Elements Boxing includes the Splitting Fist, the Crushing Fist, the Drilling Fist, the Cannon Fist, and the Crossing Fist. It is practiced in five sections.

<u>Section 1: Pi Quan (Splitting Fist)</u>

The fist called "Pi" is named for its motion, which is like an ax chopping down. When practicing, the eyes should look straight ahead or at the lead hand, the head is lifted upwards, the chest is open and expansive, the lower abdomen is filled with qi, the hips are pushed forward, the knees are slightly bent, and the two hips are tightly squeezed together. The foot follows the hand and pushes forward, with the form of the advance being like that of an arrow, straight and fast. When the foot touches the ground, the toes grip tightly to the ground and are not easily removed. The size of the step depends on the length of the body, and while the front leg has the intention of moving forward, it also has the intention of pulling back. The back leg may stand firmly, but also has the intention of moving forward. The front and back work together to create stability. The use of force in all parts should follow what was previously mentioned. When retracting the hand, the fingers should be curled like pulling a heavy object, retracting to the heart and the palm turning back into a fist. Then, it is sent out again from the heart. When the palm is retracted and turned into a fist, it contains a downward pressure. When the fist is extended, it contains an upward lift. This is because the palm is slightly higher than the heart when it is in front. When taking a large step, the back foot should be lifted to ensure a stable distance between the two feet. In the Pi fist, all steps are done with a "dian" step. In Pi fist, the hand and foot move together as one. The rest will be omitted. The technique begins from the starting position.

> (1) Clench both fists. The right arm rises up along the body with the fist facing up, extending forward from the chest to a height between the eyebrows and the neck. When the right fist has not yet passed the chest, the right arm already contains the intention to turn right, and the right thigh (from elbow to shoulder) also turns slightly. When the right fist extends from the chest, the right arm turns right with full force until the little finger of the right fist is curved into a circle facing up. At this time, the right elbow is just in front of the chest, about half a foot away from the chest, and the elbow acupoint is upward. When the right arm

moves like this, the left arm also turns left and extends forward, sticking to the front of the chest, with the fist facing up and the intention to follow the right elbow forward. At the same time, look at the right fist, raise the head up, open the chest, expand the lower abdomen, push the hips forward, slightly bend the knees, and tightly squeeze the two hips together, as shown in the first picture.

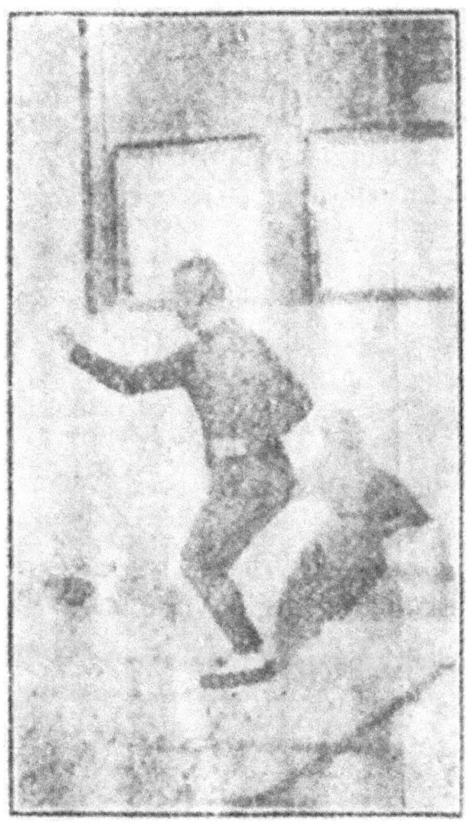

(2) The left fist extends from the heart and passes over the right elbow and arm, meeting at the point where both fists flip into palms. Both backs of the hands face upward, with the left palm slanting forward and pushing, and the right palm slanting backward and dragging, stopping at the right side of the navel. Each joint of the fingers is slightly bent, with the fingers spread apart and not touching each other, while the tiger's mouth (the space between the thumb and index finger) forms a large, rounded bend. Both palms' large, rounded bends face upward, with the left elbow tightly wrapped inside, the same as the right elbow in the first diagram, except that the first is a fist and the second is a palm. The right arm is tightly attached to the waist. When

both arms move in this way, the left foot follows the left hand's forward push and also advances. The advancing form is like an arrow, for its advance is straight and fast. When it lands, the toes hook the ground tightly, and it is firm and not easily pulled out. The size of the step depends on the length of the body. At this time, the right foot does not move, with both knees slightly bent. The left knee and the heel form a vertical line, and the right knee and the heel form a vertical line. Both legs are in a scissors-like position. The left leg in front, although with the intention of advancing, also contains the intention of later retreating, while the right leg behind, although standing still, has a somewhat forward urging intention. With the front and back sides clamping, it is stable. The use of force in all other parts follows what was mentioned before. All that is shown above can be understood by observing the second diagram. (Note: This diagram should have been facing to the left, but because the right arm cannot be seen when facing to the left, it faces to the right.)

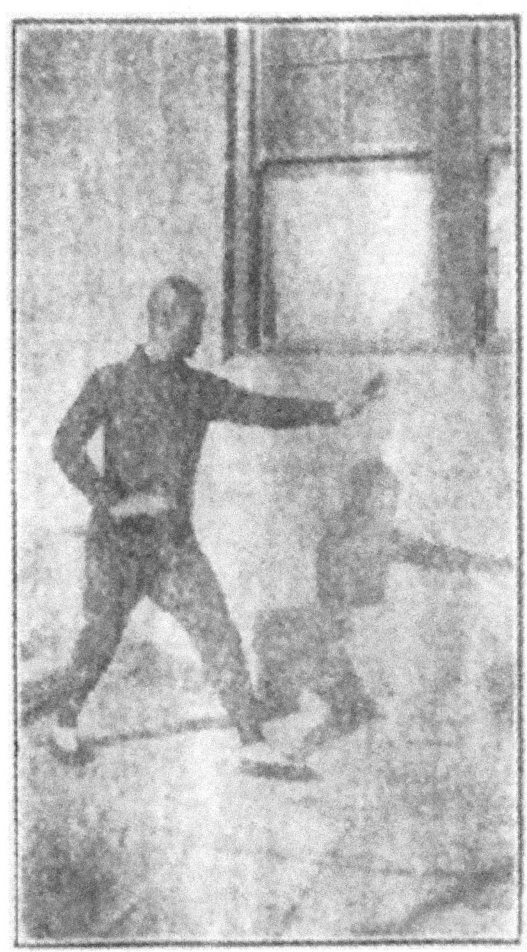

(3) The left hand retracts, using force to bend each finger like
pulling a heavy object. When it retracts to the chest, the
palm turns back into a fist. Then, it is issued from the chest,
the same as the right hand in the first figure. At the same
time, the right palm is also pulled back, transformed into a
fist and issued from the chest, the same as the left hand in
the first figure. It should be noted that when the palm is
pulled back and transformed into a fist, it contains a
downward pressure. When the fist is extended forward, it
contains an upward lifting force. This is because the fist or
palm is slightly higher than the chest at the point where it
stops in front. At the same time, the left foot goes out with
the left hand. Its stepping method is different from before.
The toe turns outward about thirty degrees, like a standing
posture, and then moves forward. It is called a "dian" step.
The back foot still steps with a "dian" step. When the front
foot takes a big step, the back foot steps up to maintain a

fixed distance between the two feet to avoid instability. In the "Pi Quan" (splitting fist) form, all steps that follow the fist are "dian" steps. This section describes the "Pi Quan" form as shown in the third figure.

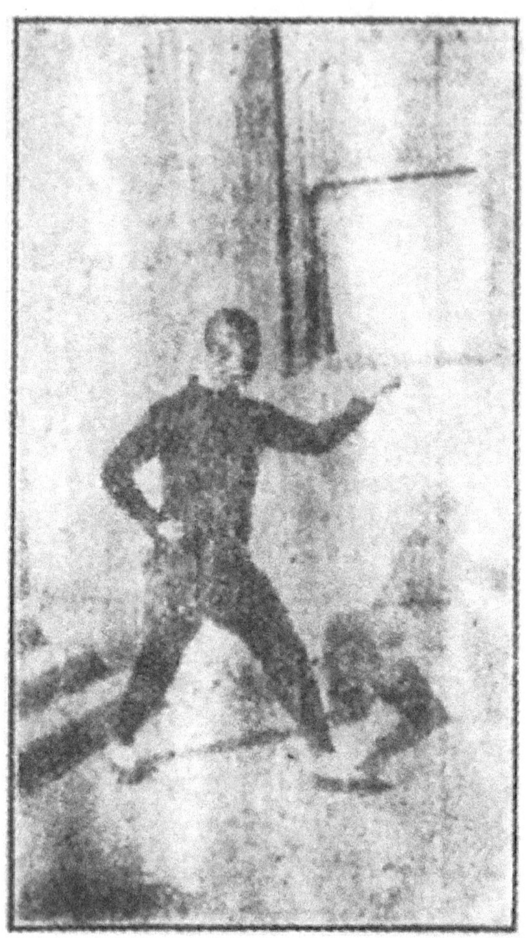

(4) Then the right hand and right foot move forward. The right hand changes into a palm, performing the same movement as the left hand and left foot in the second picture. This section describes the palm technique of the Splitting Fist, as shown in the fourth picture.

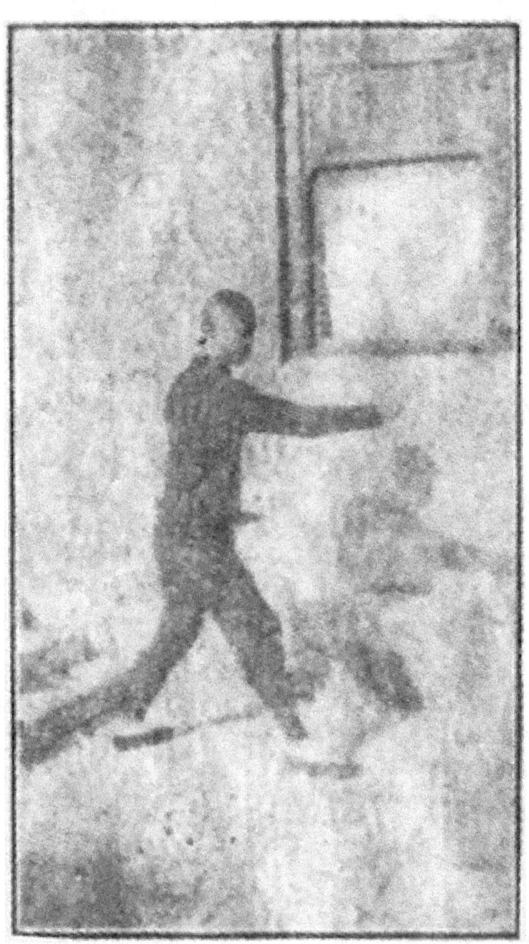

(5) The movement of the right hand and right foot is the same as that of the left hand and left foot in the third picture.

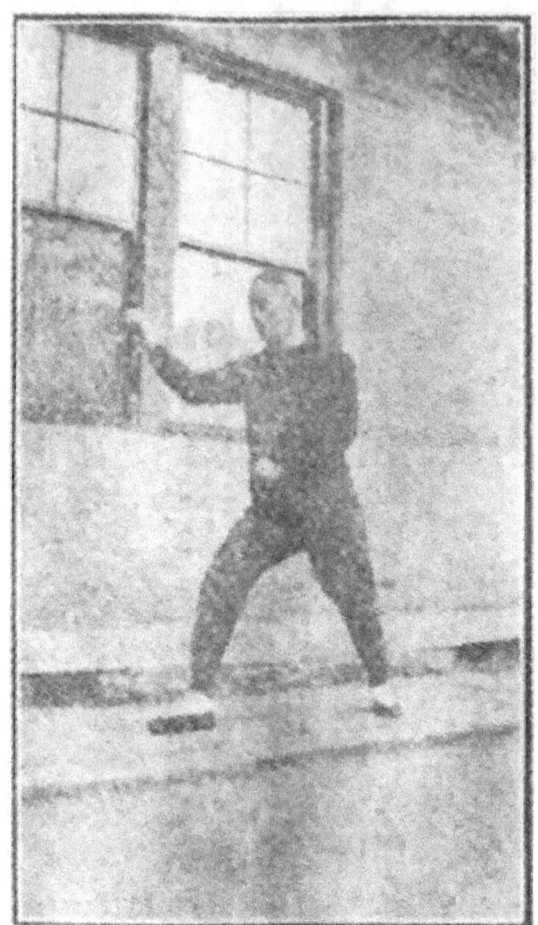

(6) The movement of the left hand and left foot is the same as in the second diagram. The left hand changes back into a palm.

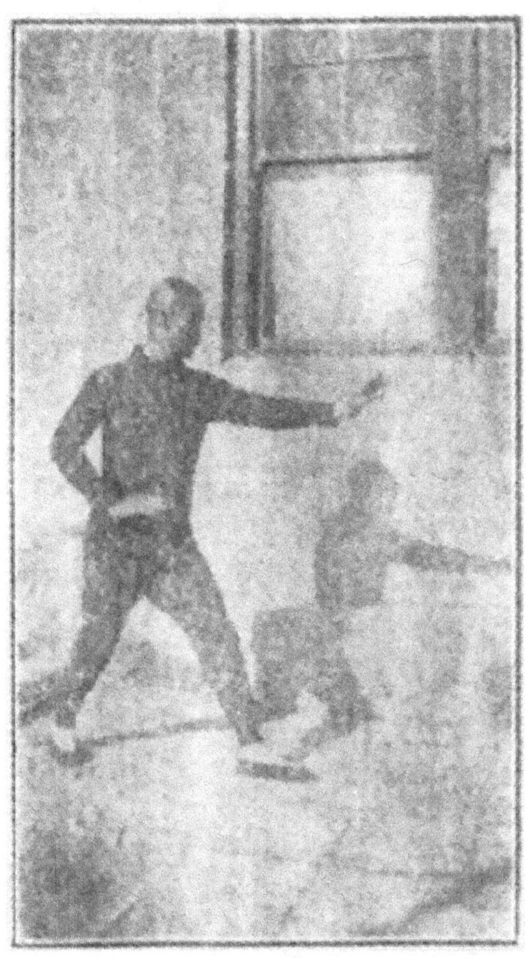

In this way, the movements continue without interruption. Whenever one hand changes into a palm, it becomes a Pi Quan (Splitting Fist). To execute a left Pi Quan, the right fist and right foot must be forward. To execute a right Pi Quan, the left fist and left foot must be forward. To turn around, when the left hand performs the Pi Quan, one must turn to the right and become the right foot and right hand forward. When the right hand performs the fist, it is the same as the previous movement to perform the Pi Quan. When the right hand performs the Pi Quan, one must turn to the left and take advantage of the momentum. In Pi Quan, the hands and feet should follow each other. If the left hand is in front, the left foot is also in front, and the right hand is in the back, the right foot is also in the back. After becoming proficient, the fist and palm movements can be combined into one movement. When using the fist movement, the back foot does not need to follow and stop, and the palm movement can be directly performed by advancing forward.

<u>Section 2: Beng Quan (Crushing Fist)</u>

The meaning of "Beng" is the collapse of a mountain, which is
extremely powerful. This fist is similar in nature, hence its name. It
is important to note that the right elbow must be wrapped inward,
like in the Pi fist. This ensures that the elbow acupoint points
upwards and slightly downwards, so that the entire body does not
become stiff. This is the subtlety of the technique, and it can be
achieved through long-term practice (see Chapter 6). The toes
should shoot straight forward, and the right foot can be extended to
touch the root of the left foot to enhance the momentum. At the
same time, the body should be straight and the head should not
droop. The leg must be slightly bent to avoid taking too small of a
step. The starting position is the same as the first and second
diagrams of the "Pi Quan". The first move is a "piquan" palm
strike.

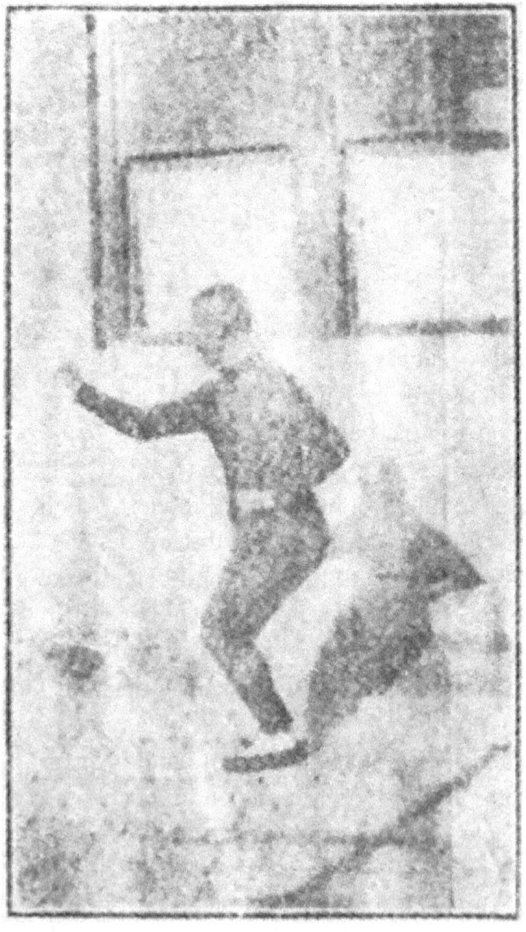

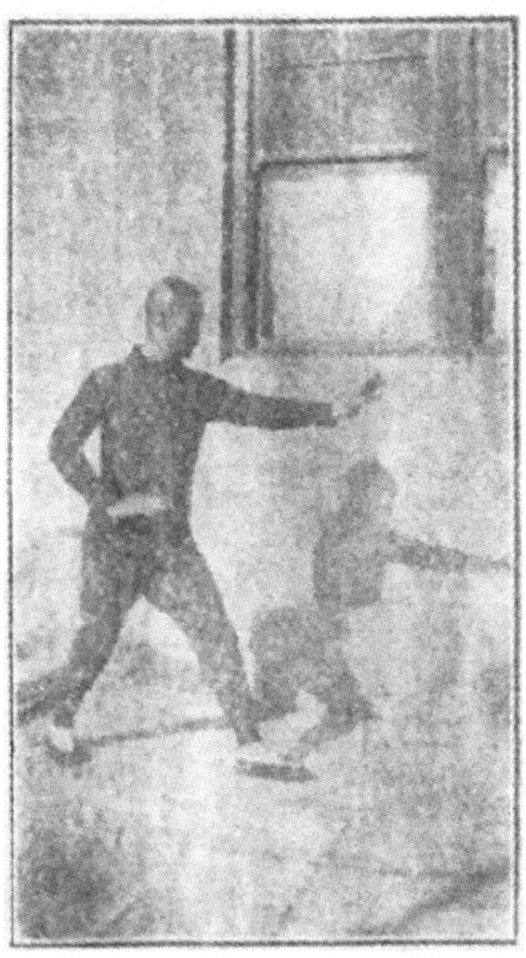

(1) When performing the Pi Quan posture, the left hand in front and the right hand in the back transform into fists at the same time, with the index and middle fingers forming a circle pointing upwards for the left hand, and the fist facing upwards for the right hand. Then the left fist is pulled back and placed at the waist, with the fist turning upwards during the withdrawal, while the right fist is extended from the heart and turns sideways, transforming into the left fist stance that has just been in front. Learners should pay attention to wrapping the right elbow inward as in Pi Quan, so that the elbow point tilts slightly downward and avoids stiffness throughout the body. This is a wonderful skill that can be acquired through long practice (see Chapter 6). At the same time, the left foot follows the front strike of the right fist and steps forward, with the foot pointing straight ahead. Then the right foot follows with a shuffle step, which should be smaller than the Pi Quan step. The right

foot can even touch the left foot to enhance the force. The body should be straight with the head upright and not drooping. The leg must be slightly tilted because the step is small. The leg stance is the same as in the first diagram of Pi Quan. For more clarity, refer to the fifth diagram.

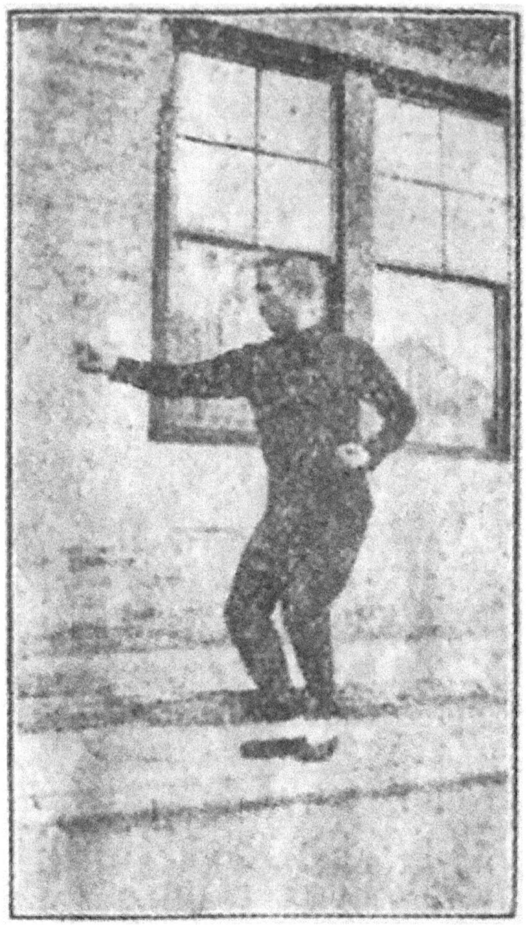

(2) Then the left fist is released and the right fist is withdrawn, the technique is the same as in the fifth diagram. However, regardless of which fist is in front, the left foot is always in front and the right foot always follows from behind. As shown in the sixth diagram.

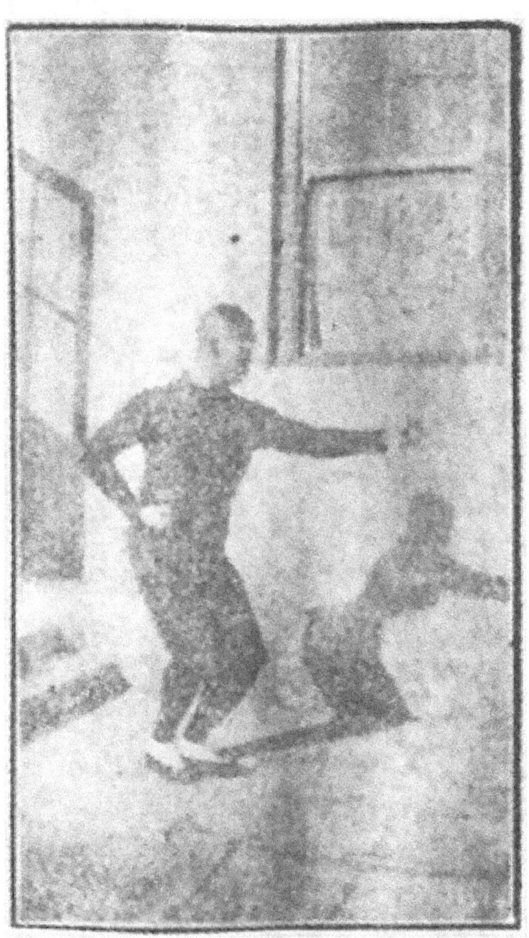

(3) When turning, turn from the right side. After turning, the
    right fist makes the fist posture of the splitting fist. The
    right leg is lifted, and the sole of the foot faces outward to
    step on the opponent, as shown in the seventh picture.

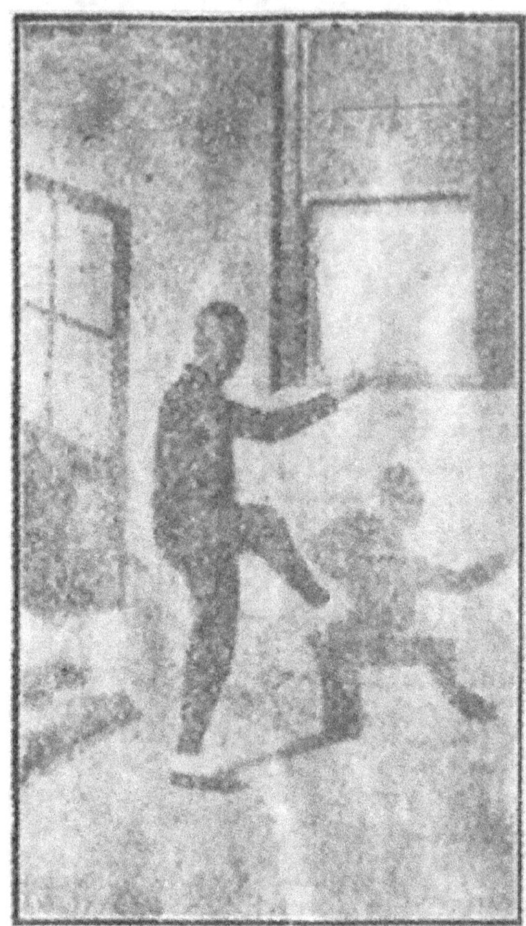

(4) Then assume the palm position of Pi Quan. The left hand pushes forward, the right hand retracts backward, and the right leg falls in front of the left foot, with the right foot forming a straight line. Like the eighth picture.

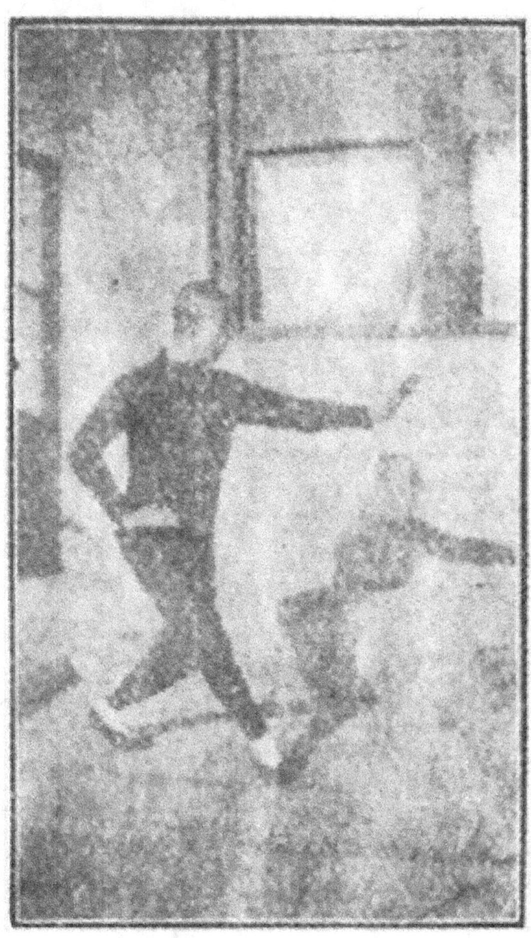

(5) Then the left foot and right fist are sent forward, same as in
the fifth picture.

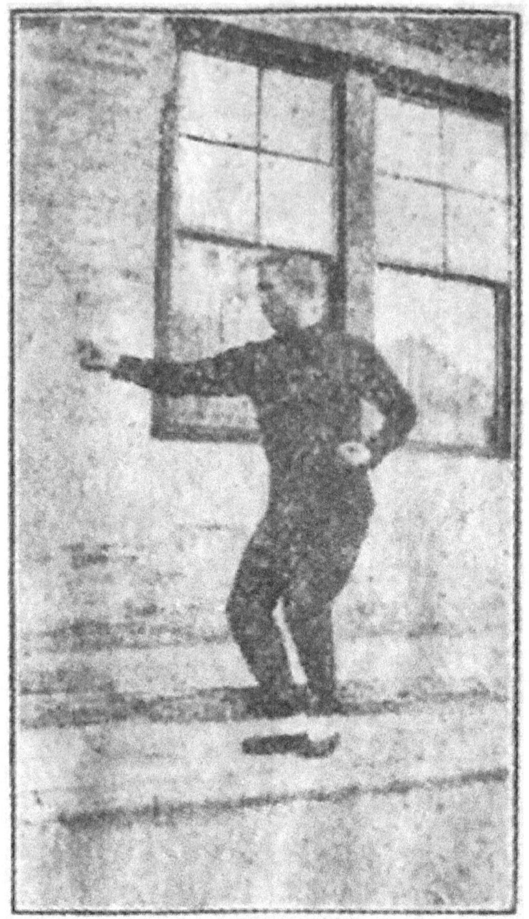

Continuously repeat this sequence, whenever turning, always turn to the right so that the left foot remains in the front and it is inconvenient to turn to the left.

<u>Section 3: Zuan Quan (Drilling Fist)</u>

The meaning of "zuan" is to concentrate force. This technique's movements resemble the action of drilling, hence the name "zuan quan." The initial movements of this technique are the same as in the first and second images of the piquan technique, beginning with the fist position and palm position of the splitting technique.

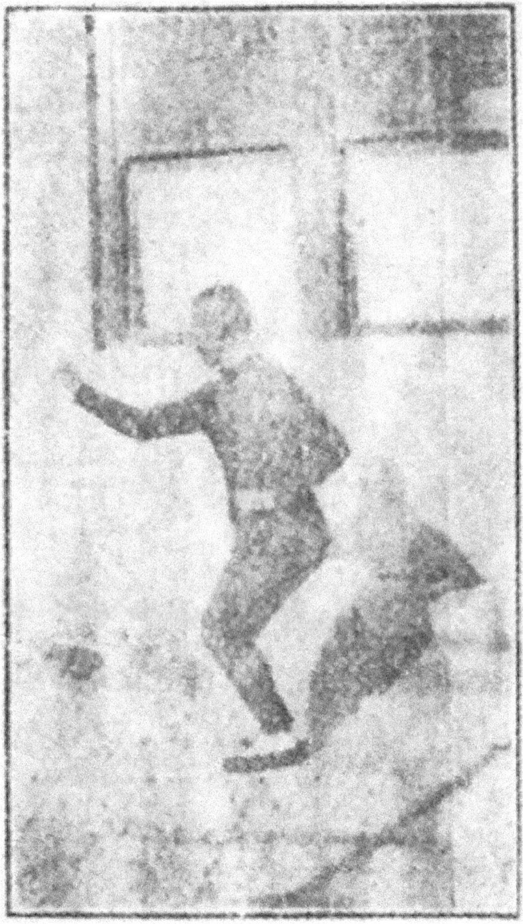

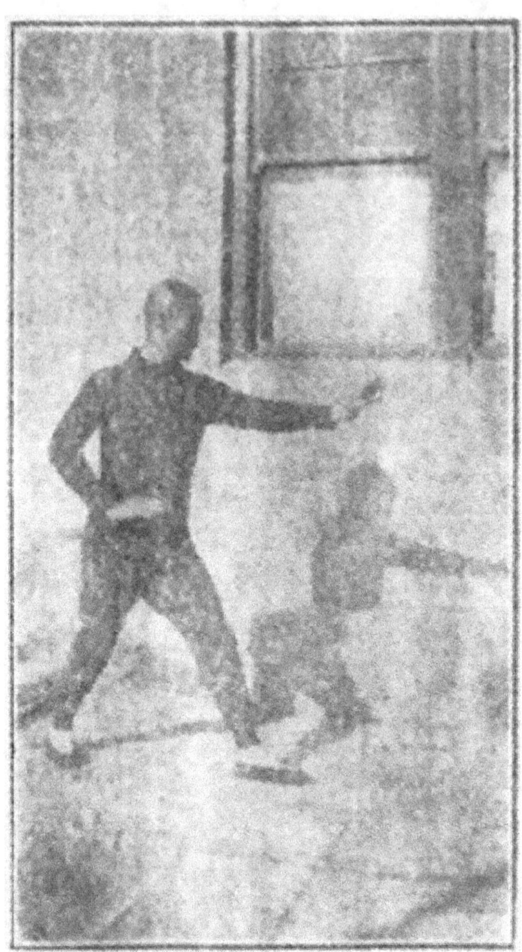

(1) Both palms turn into fists. The left fist is positioned with the back of the fist facing upwards in front, while the right fist is positioned likewise behind. The left fist has a downward pressure while the right fist is ready to extend forward. At the same time, the left foot in front steps forward, and the right foot behind follows, using the same footwork as the chop fist. See Figure 9. (Note: the back of the left fist has not turned upwards in this figure.)

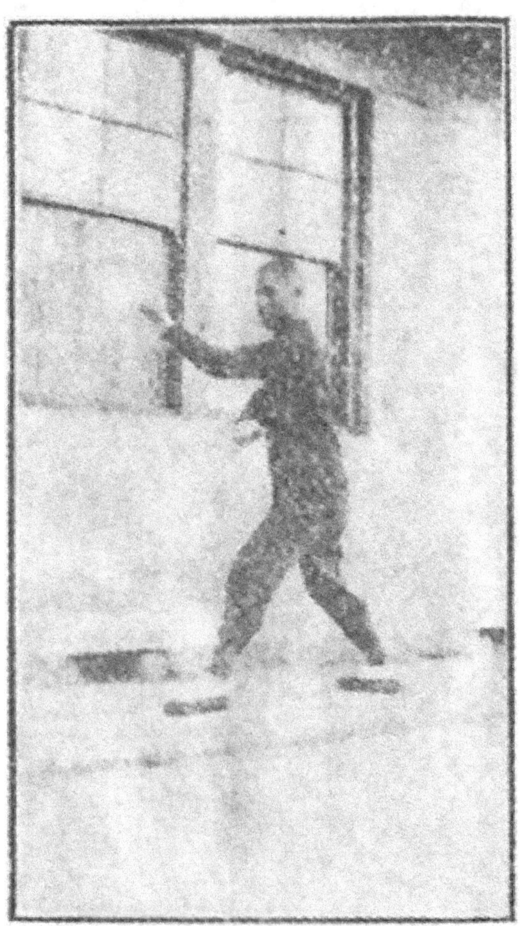

(2) Then the left arm presses down and withdraws, while the right fist strikes up towards the left arm, using the same technique as the Splitting Fist. The left arm stops at the left side of the navel, close to the body, with the back of the fist facing upwards. At the same time, the right foot follows the right fist out, with the left foot immediately following. The footwork is the same as that of the Splitting Fist palm. The size of the steps can be adjusted as needed. See Figure 10.

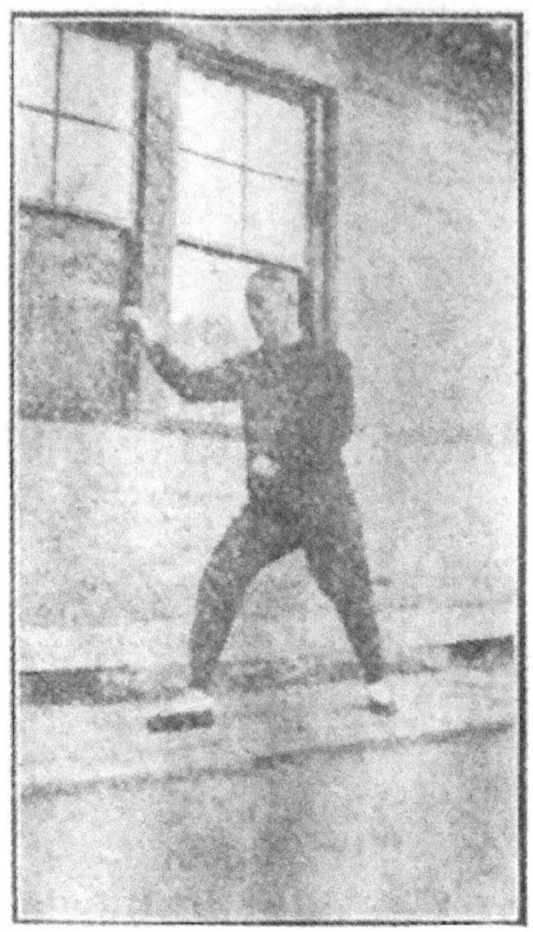

(3) When the left fist strikes out, it imitates the previous movement.

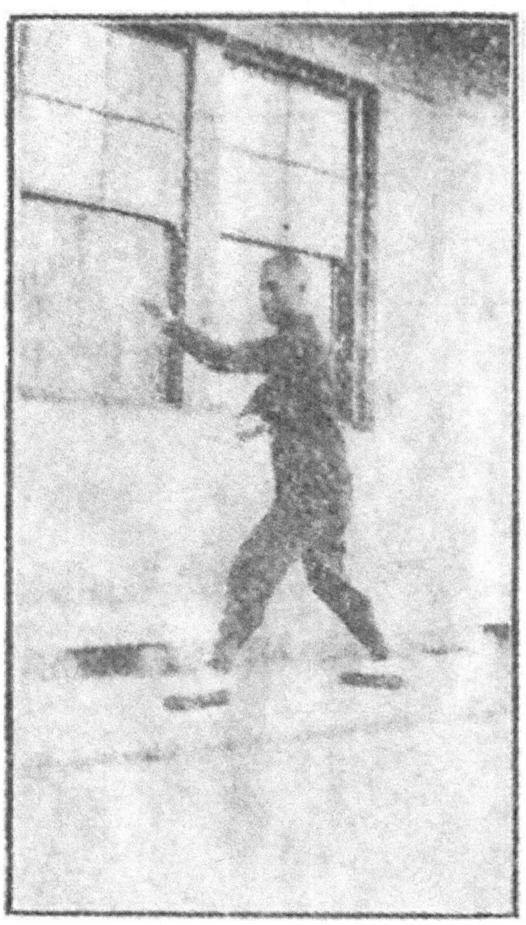

(4) There are two ways to turn the body.
    a.   Same as the splitting fist.
    b.   If the left hand and left foot are in front, turn to the right to switch the right foot to the front. During the turn, the left fist extends forward, presses down, and then withdraws. Then, the right fist takes the opportunity to strike upward from the position of the left fist. After the turn, the right foot is in front, and immediately advances with the strike of the right fist. The left foot follows. This is shown in the eleventh picture.

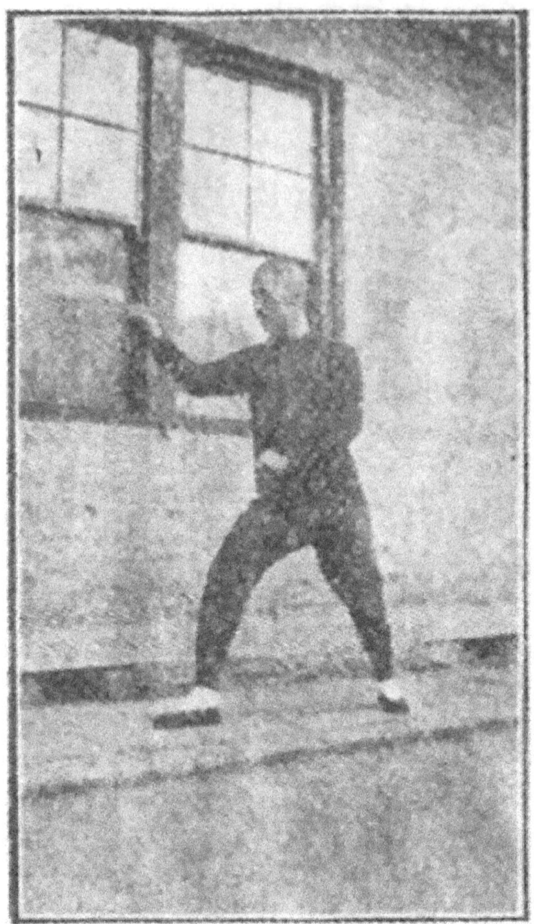

This method is extremely wonderful. When the enemy attacks from behind, I can use one fist to press down their attacking fist while at the same time my right fist strikes their face. After practicing, (one) and (two) can be combined into one move. That is, when performing the first move, the left foot advances and the right foot does not need to follow and stop, and can immediately continue with the second move.

<u>Section 4: Pao Quan (Cannon Fist)</u>

The meaning of "pao" is similar to "beng", which means that the action of the fist is like that of a cannon. This fist is used to break the enemy from high to low. The essence of Xingyi is that when attacking the enemy, you can also defend yourself at the same time. When the enemy attacks me and I defend myself, I can also attack the enemy. Therefore, people often cannot defend themselves in time. Both legs are slightly bent, the right leg has a forward thrust, and the left leg in front also has a stable standing intention. At the same time, the qi of the whole body is gathered in the lower abdomen and secretly transported to the limbs. The strength of the two arms, which was originally not much, must be increased several times. Because of the increased strength, even a strong man cannot withstand it. It begins with the splitting technique.

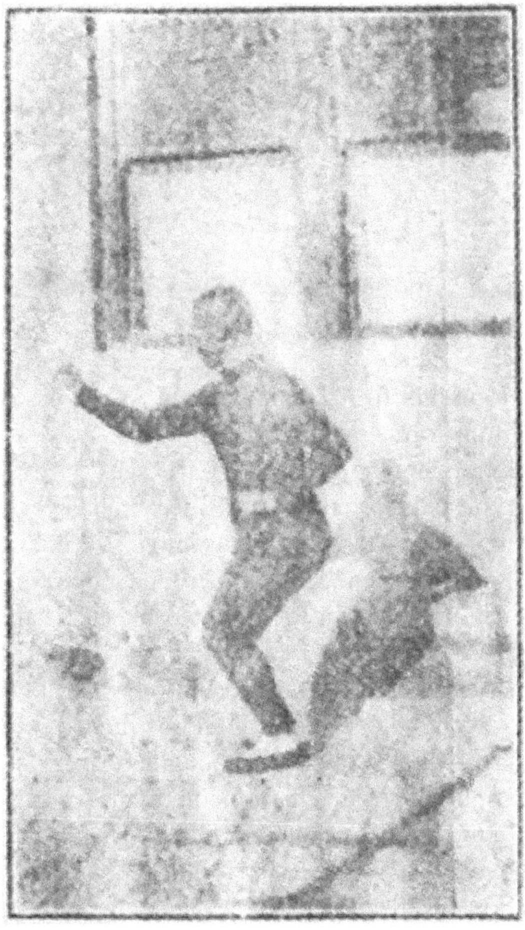

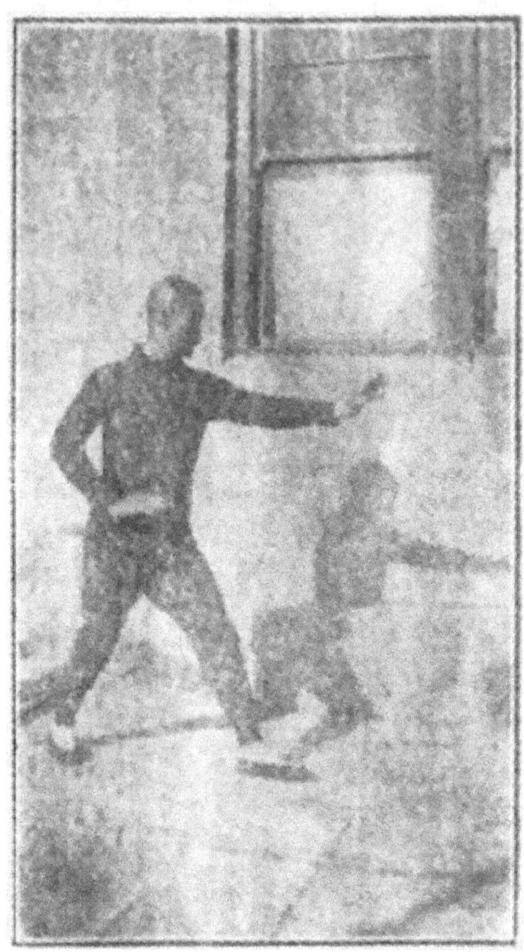

(1) Both palms transform into fists simultaneously. When the left palm in front transforms into a fist, it is immediately retracted. When retracting, the back of the fist faces downwards and is placed close to the left side of the navel. After the right palm in the back transforms into a fist, it is also facing downwards, placed close to the right side of the navel. At the same time, the right foot in the back steps half forward to the right, and the left foot immediately follows up. The right side of the left foot should be close to the left side of the right foot, and the left foot should be lifted slightly without touching the ground. Although the body is half facing to the right, the head is half facing to the left. Like in the twelfth picture. (Explanation: the left foot does not necessarily have to be attached to the right foot as the book says to connect this posture with the following posture, but in the picture, it has to be separated into two postures.)

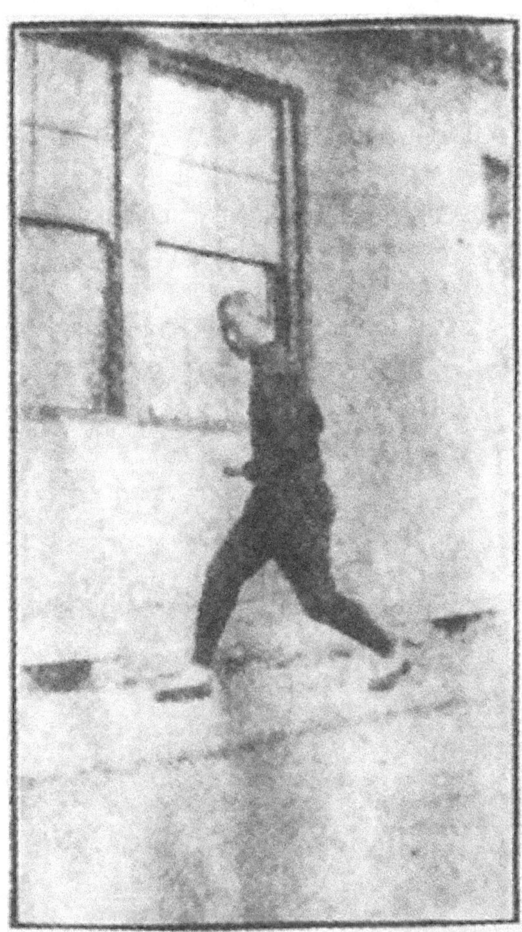

(2) The left fist rises close to the body, with the back of the fist
facing downwards. Suddenly, when it reaches the face, it
rotates and the inside of the fist faces outwards. The back
of the fist stops in front of the forehead without touching it.
When it rotates, the whole arm uses force to push outward
and upward, this fist can break the enemy's fist when they
are striking down from high. At the same time, the right
hand immediately does a bengquan and strikes in the
direction of the head, the enemy is hit by my fist. This is
the essence of Xingyi. When you strike at the enemy, you
can protect yourself at the same time. When the enemy
strikes me and I protect myself, I can also strike the enemy
immediately. Therefore, the enemy cannot defend in time.
However, this is still not the most wonderful thing. At this
time, my left foot, which does not touch the ground, takes
advantage of this and steps forward in an arrow step
towards the direction of the right hand strike. The right foot

follows from behind. The stepping method is like that of bengquan. Both legs are slightly bent. The right leg has the force of pushing forward, while the left leg in front is stable. At the same time, gather the qi of the whole body in the lower abdomen and secretly move it to the limbs. Then, the power of the two arms, which was not much before, must be increased several times. With this several-fold increase in power, even a strong man cannot withstand it. See picture 13.

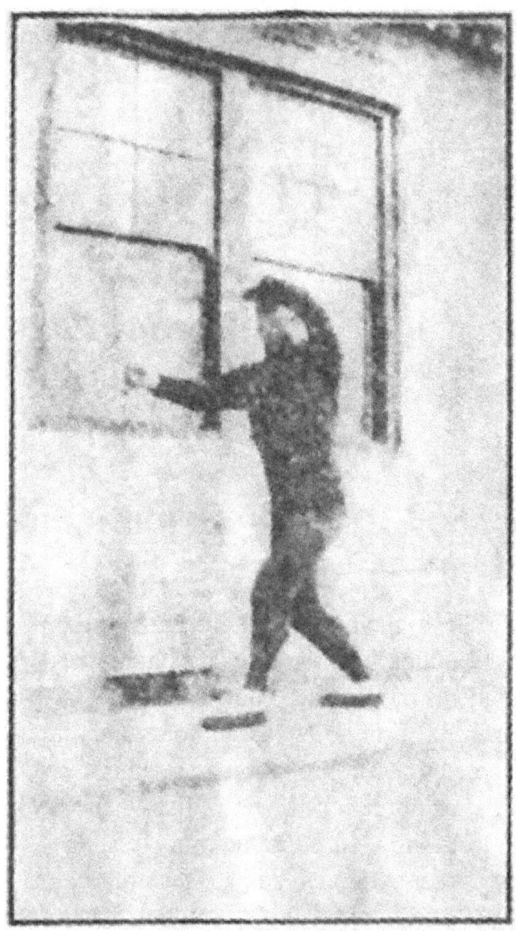

(3) At present, the body is half-turned to the left. The left foot in front is still moving forward in this direction. The right foot follows, lifts up and rests beside the left foot. Both fists are lowered and placed on both sides of the navel, the same as (1). Refer to Figure 14.

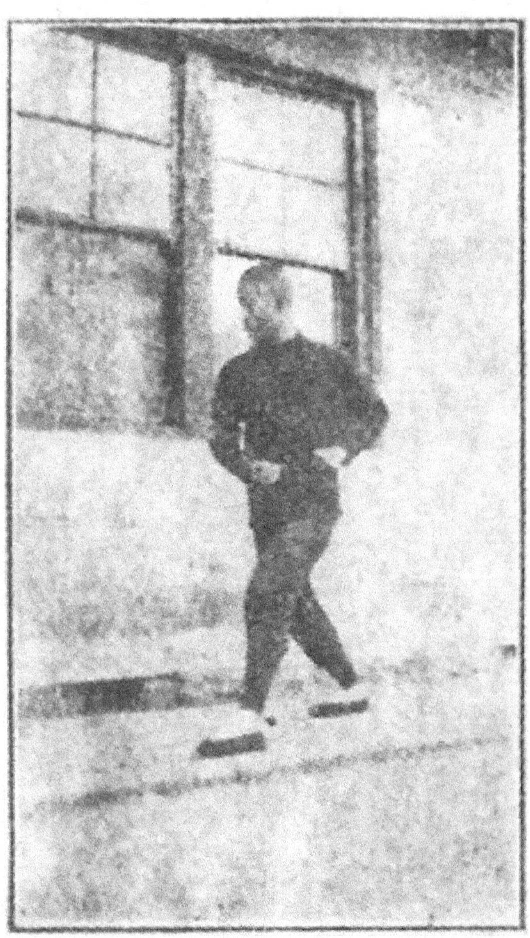

(4) The right fist turns upward and outward. The left fist performs a Beng Quan punch. The raised right foot follows the punch forward to the right. The left foot follows. This is the same as (2). See picture 15.

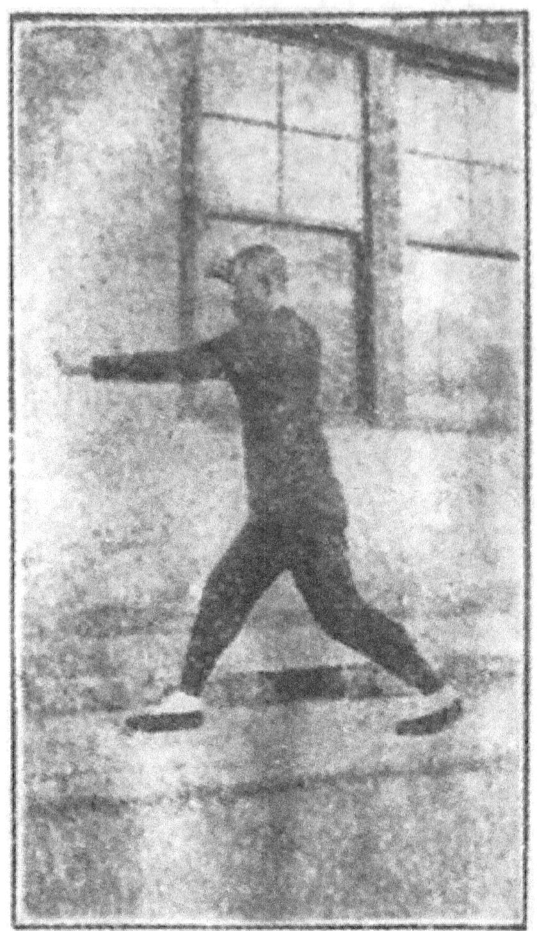

In this way, it continues without interruption. When turning around, if the body is half turned to the left, the left leg hooks to the right, and the body turns to the back. The right foot still follows, lifts up, and leans against the left foot. As in picture 16. (Note) This picture is similar to picture 14, except that the direction is different. The former moves forward while the latter turns back, but the form is the same.

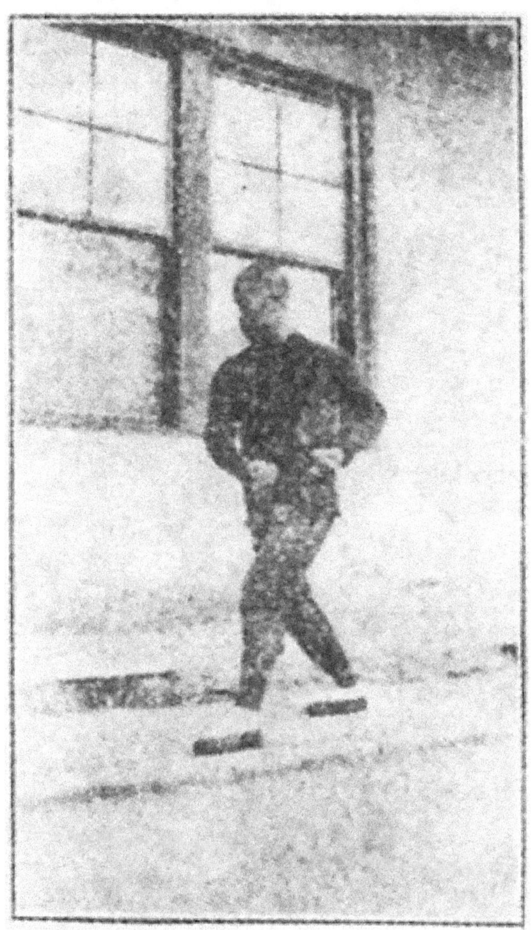

Then the right foot and left fist are launched, similar to before. The direction of the forward step is clear from the seventeenth picture. The direction of the forward step for the crossing fist is also the same.

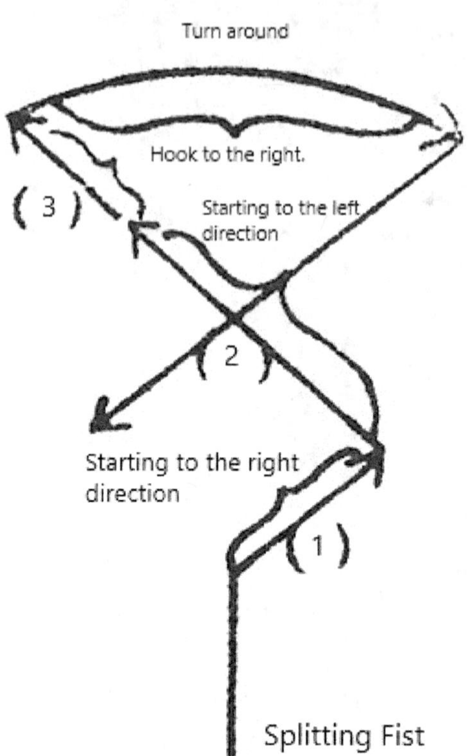


Splitting Fist

<u>Section 5: Heng Quan (Crossing Fist)</u>

The application of this fist is not straight but horizontal, hence its name, "crossing fist". When practicing, the elbow should be tightly wrapped and the back fist should be released from under the elbow of the forearm. Remember this. It begins with a splitting fist posture.

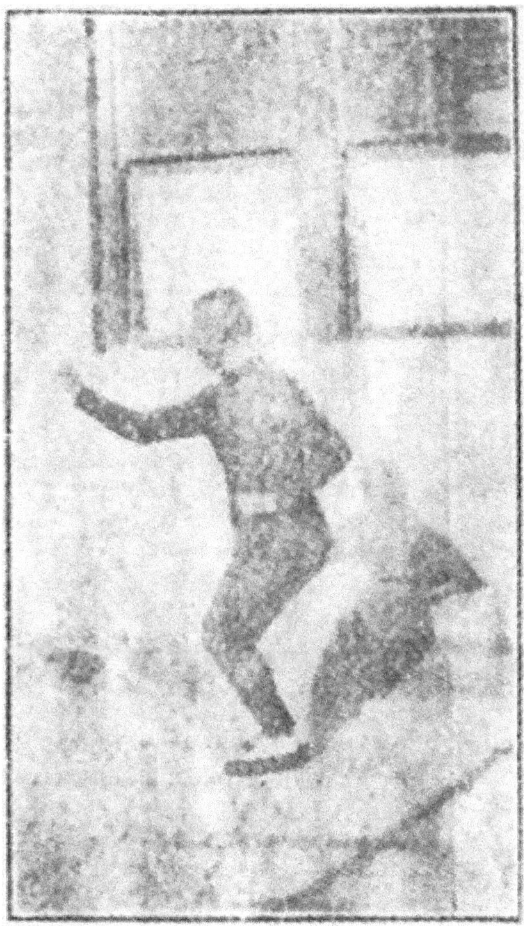

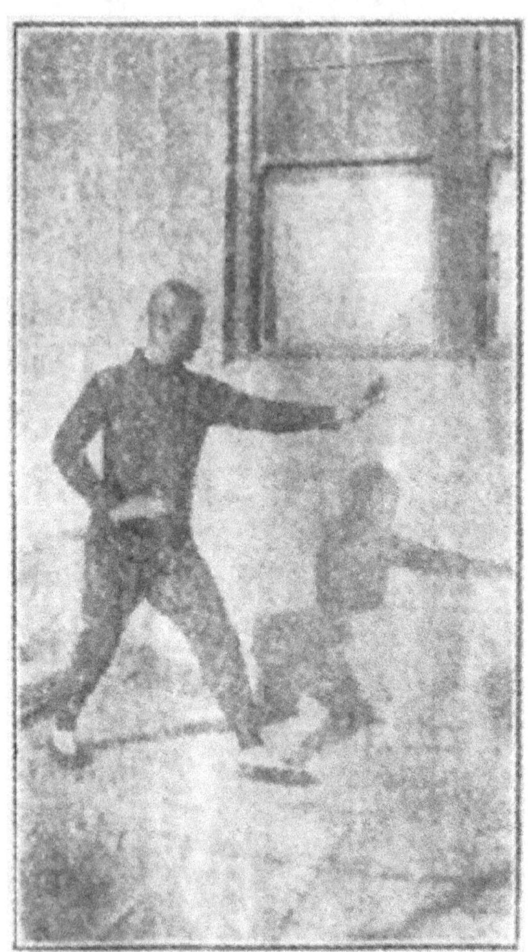

(1) Step forward with the right foot from behind, left foot
follows and lifts up, the same as cannon punch. (Note:
students must remember that the footwork for crossing fist
and cannon punch are the same.) At the same time, the
palm changes to a fist. When the left palm becomes a fist in
front, the fist's center is turned upwards, still in front, and
the elbow is tightly wrapped. When the right palm becomes
a fist from behind, the back of the hand is still facing
upwards. The rest is the same as cannon punch. See picture
18.

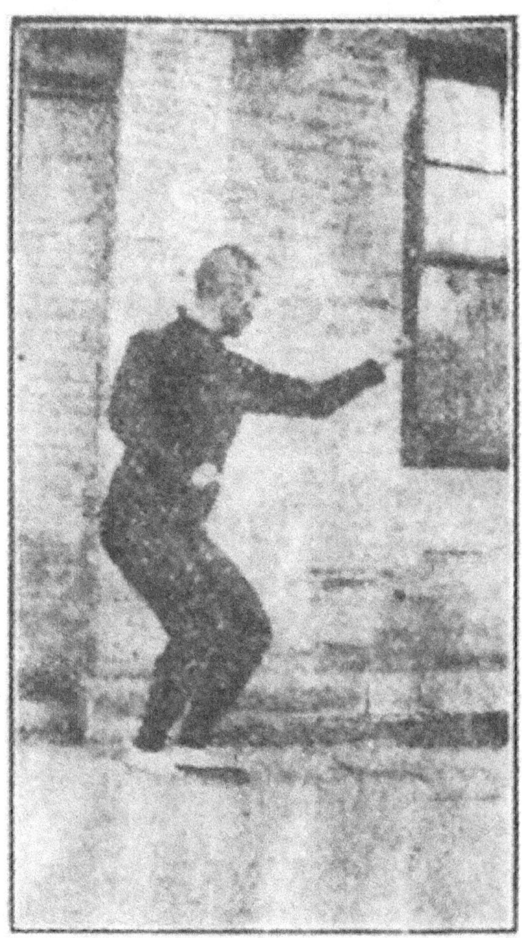

(2) The right fist is released from under the left elbow, and thrusts towards the left front. Just as the fist passes the elbow, the body turns and the fist center faces upward, with the elbow tightly wrapped, similar to the "Cannon Punch". At the same time, the left fist is withdrawn and placed close to the left side of the navel. The left foot, which was just lifted, then shoots forward to the left as an arrow step, which is exactly the same as the "Cannon Punch". See Picture 19.

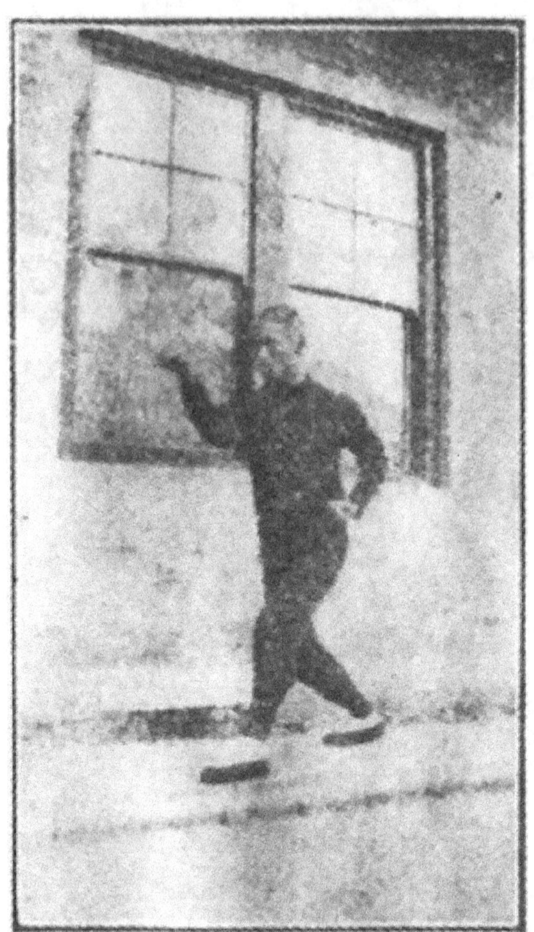

(3) Left foot steps forward. Fist doesn't move. (Later, before throwing the cross fist, one must first step forward with the front foot to synchronize the movements of hands and feet and prevent confusion.) Then, the left fist strikes out with a twist punch from under the right elbow to the right front. The right fist is retracted. At the same time, the right foot steps forward to the right front. This is shown in Picture 20.

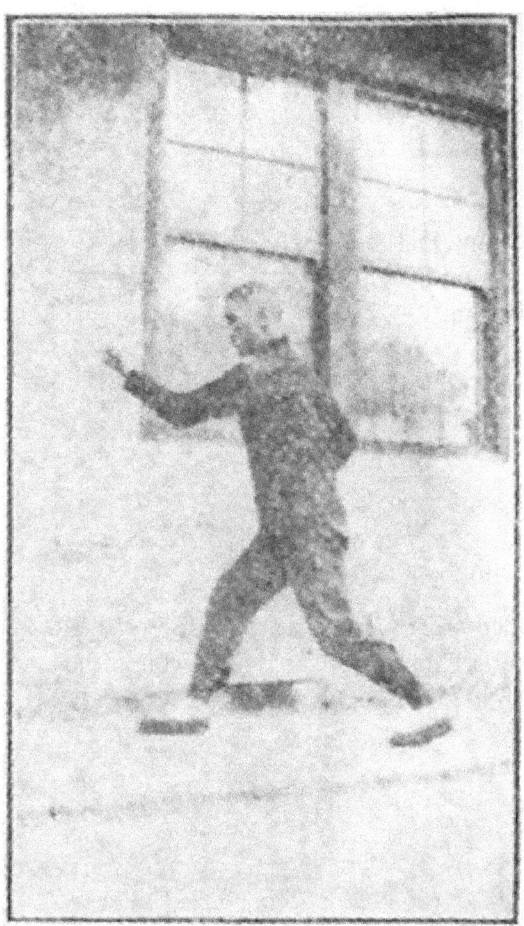

In this way, the movements continue one after another without interruption. When turning, follow the same method as for the Cannon Fist. However, when hooking the leg and turning, the fist does not move. Only after the leg has hooked and the body has turned, the fist is sent out from below the elbow.

"Continuous Advancing and Retreating Boxing" is a set of five consecutive punches. There are eleven moves in total.

1. Splitting Fist
2. Crushing Fist
3. Retreating Crushing Fist
4. Advancing Crushing Fist
5. Double Crossing Fists
6. Cannon Fist
7. Retreating Chopping Fist
8. Splitting Fist
9. Drilling Fist
10. Splitting Fist
11. Crushing Fist
12. Perform a Crushing Fist and Turning

Then repeat the sequence in the same order as before. When performing the Retreating Crushing Fist for the second time, end the sequence and return to the starting position.

### (1) Pi Quan (Splitting Fist)

Like in picture 21.

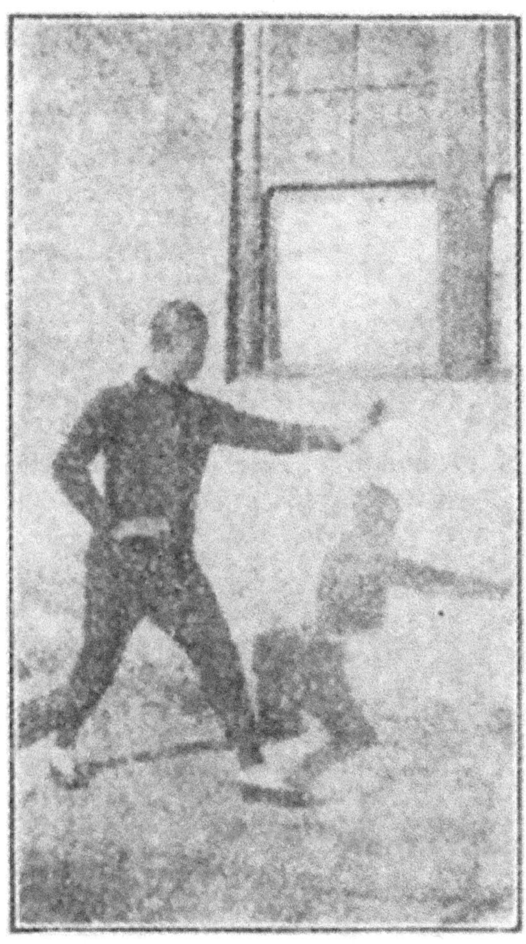

## (2) Beng Quan (Crushing Fist)

Like the 22nd picture.

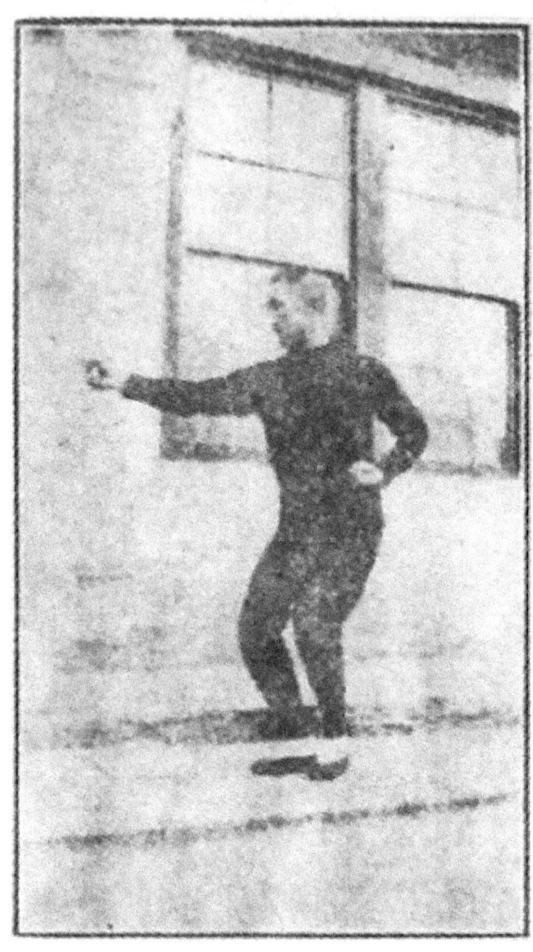

## (3) Retreating Crushing Fist

The method is to first step back with the right foot behind, then the left foot steps back one step behind the right foot. At the same time, the right fist is retracted and the left fist is sent out. This is shown in the 23rd picture.

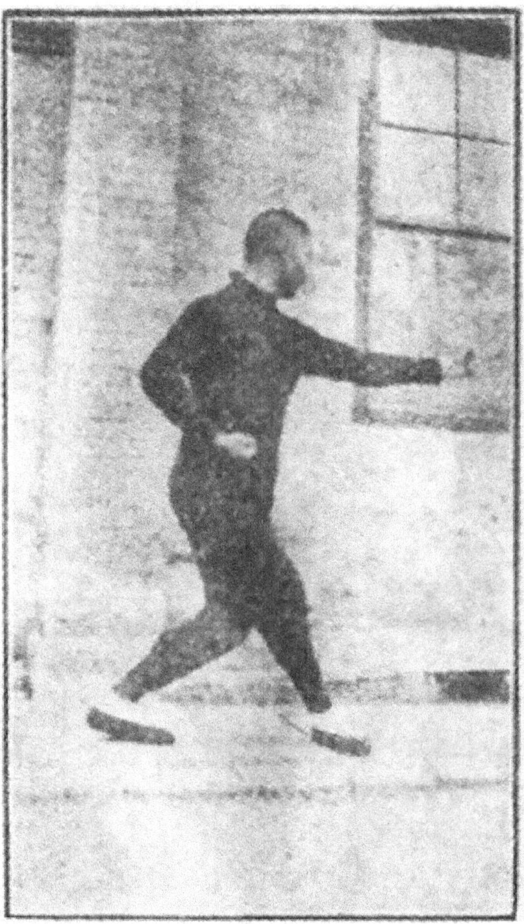

(4) Forward-step Crushing Fist

The " Forward step Crushing Fist " refers to the right foot and right fist, or the left foot and left fist, moving forward together. It is not appropriate to have the left foot move forward from behind while the right fist strikes at the same time, so the right foot that is in front should move forward with the right fist simultaneously. At the same time, the left fist is retracted, and the left foot catches up. This is shown in the 24th picture.

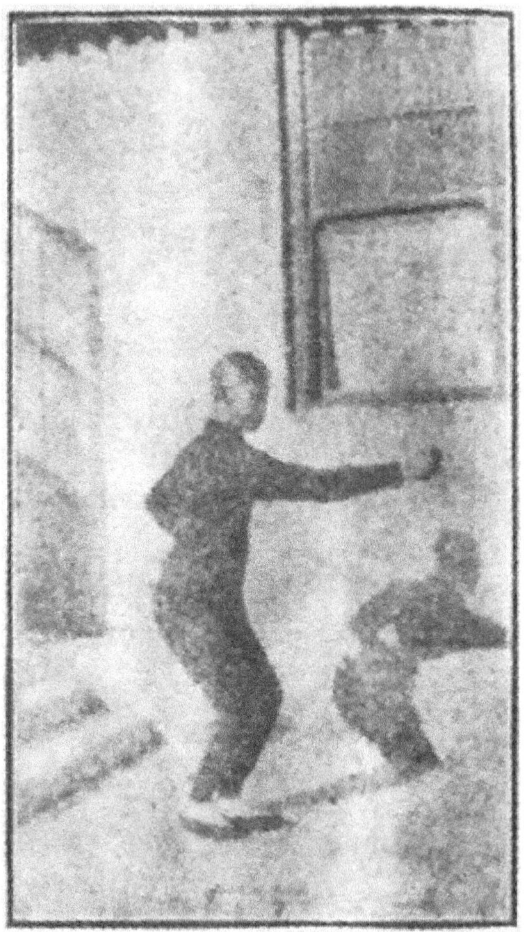

### (5) Double Crossing Fists

Two fists intersect, with the right fist on the outside. The body is half facing left. Like in Picture 25.

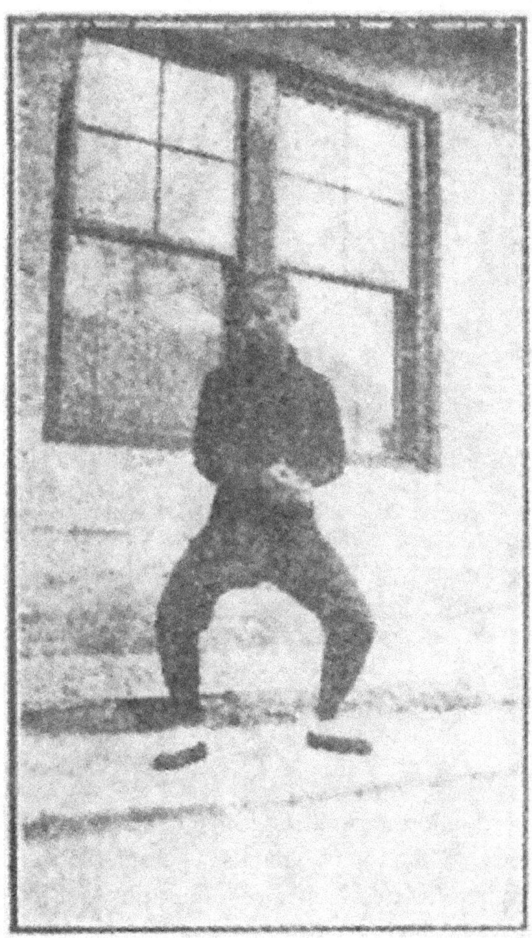

Then, the two fists separate. Both arms make a half-circle bend, not stiff and straight, but still slightly bent with power, as shown in Picture 26.

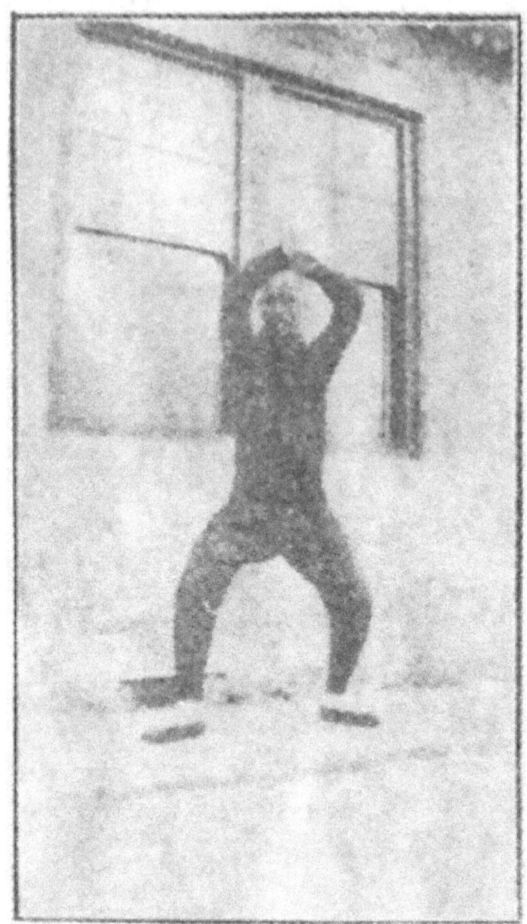

Then the left fist is released, and the right fist joins the left fist at the navel, close to the body. When the two hands separate, the left foot behind steps back. When the two hands join, the right foot in front aligns with the left foot. The body still faces half to the left, as shown in Picture 27. (Note) The difference is that the two feet in the lower part of this figure should be aligned as mentioned in the book.

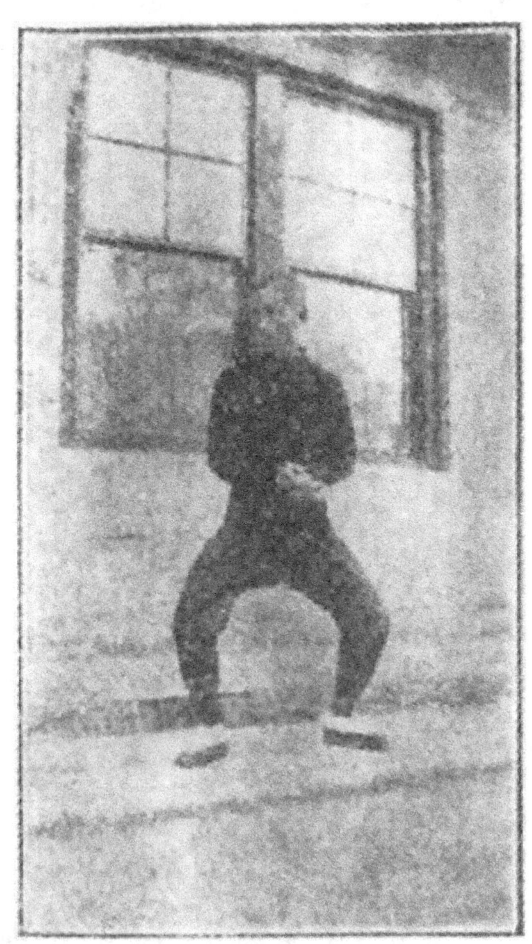

(6) Pao Quan

Make a left fist with the right foot forward, this is the Pao Quan.
As shown in Figure 28.

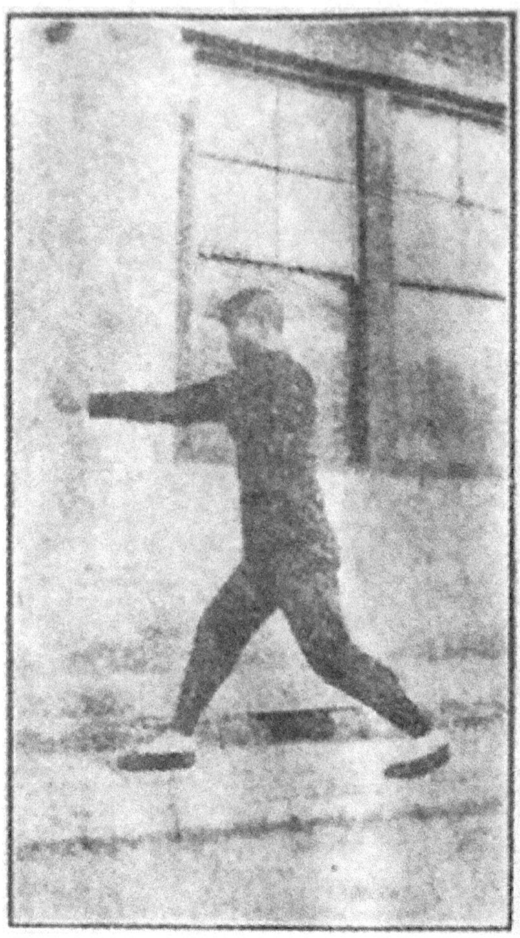

## (7) Retreating Splitting Fist

Begin by retreating the right foot. As the right fist falls down, it makes a half-circle forward. The left fist must be withdrawn first, and then chopped out again. At the same time, the left foot should slightly retreat, staying in front of the right foot. This is shown in the 29th picture.

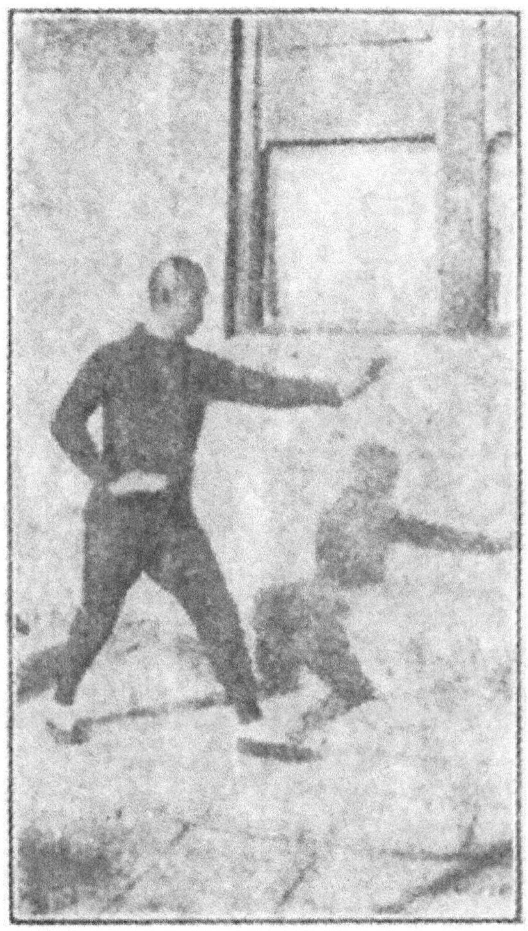

(8) Splitting Fist

However, the left hand and left foot should still be in front for this splitting fist. The method is to first turn the left palm in front into a fist and pull it back to the chest, then chop out from the chest. At the same time, the right hand that is close to the body also changes from a fist to a palm. Like in the 30th picture.

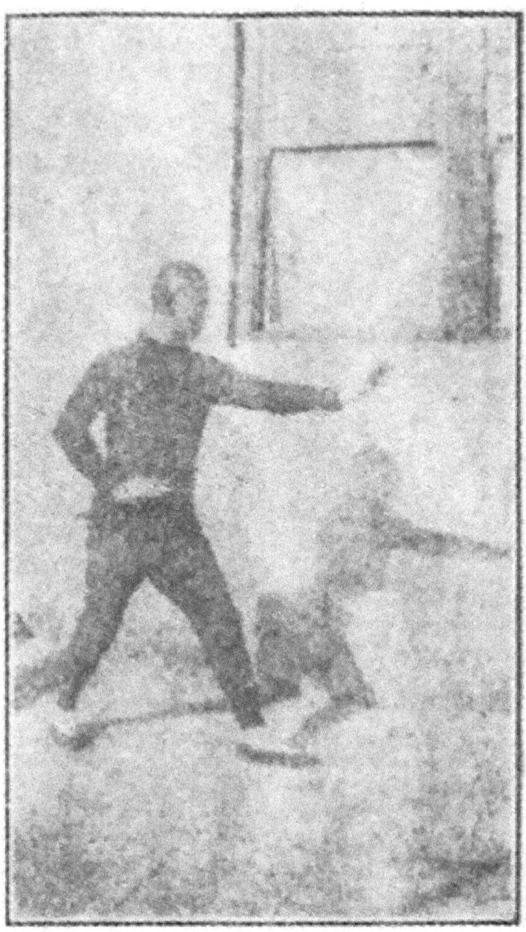

(9) Drilling Fist

The right hand and left foot are in front, as shown in figure 31.

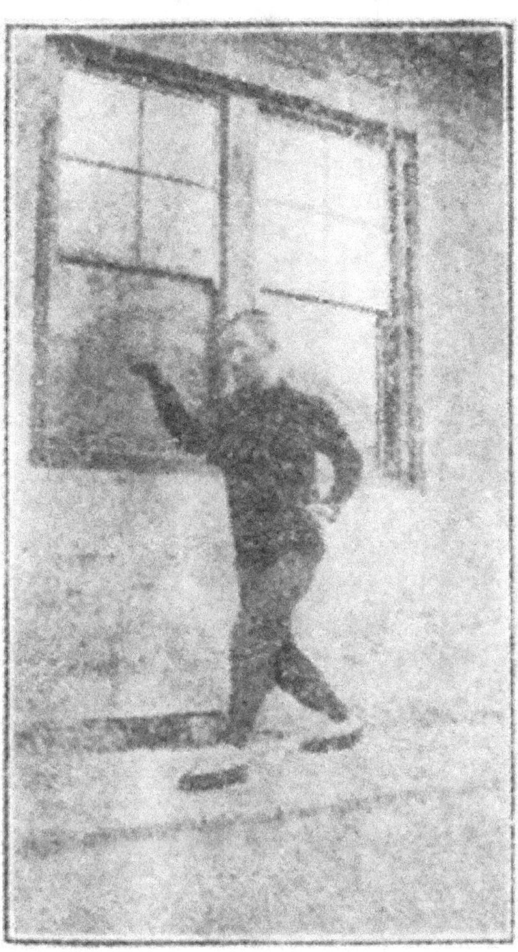

(10) Splitting Fist

Left hand and right foot in front, as shown in Figure 32.

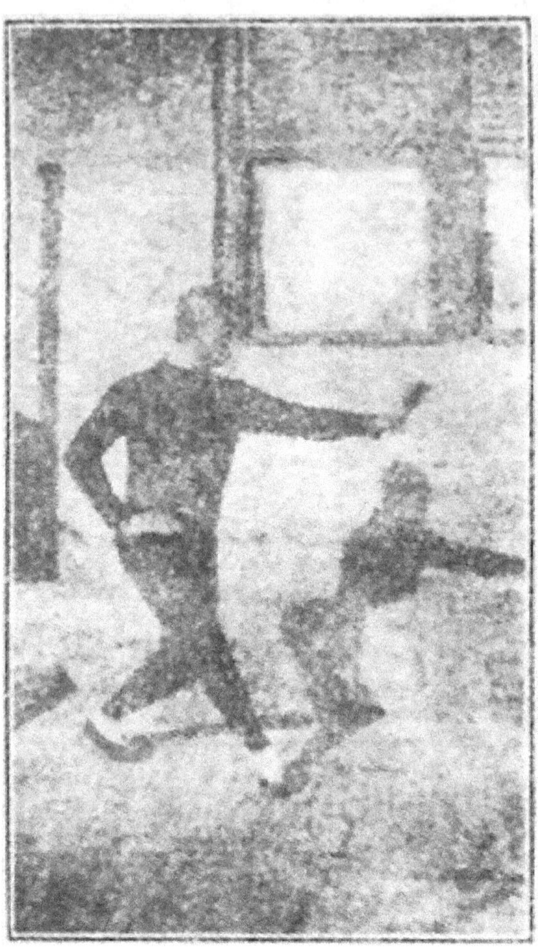

(11) Crushing Fist

Like the image shown in Picture 33.

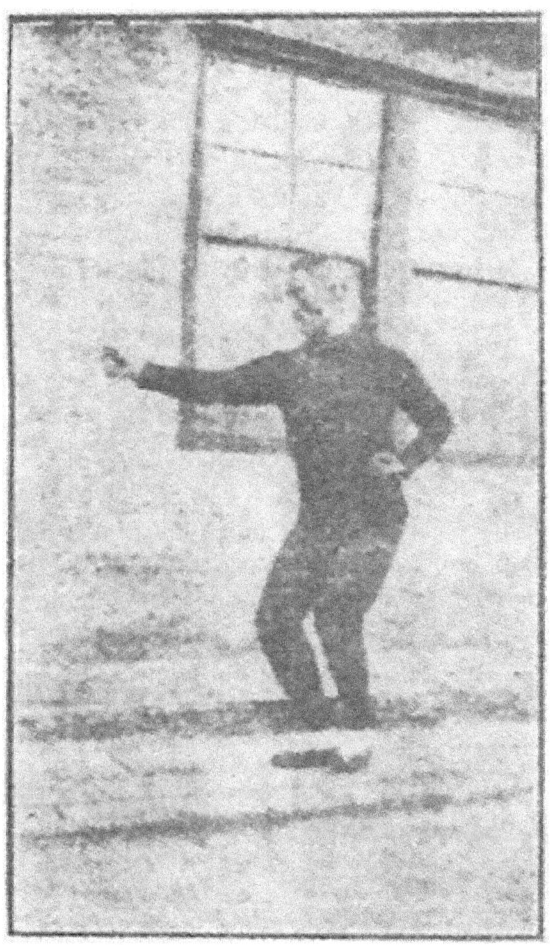

(12) Perform a Crushing Fist and turn the body.

After the turn, the sequence remains the same as before. Stop after performing the retreat smashing punch, which is used to finish the form.

# Chapter 5: The Profound Meaning of Xingyi Quan

Form refers to the posture, which can be seen by others, while intention refers to the focus of the mind. The mind is not visible to others but controls the form. The form cannot move on its own. The movement of the form is mostly controlled by the mind. The heart, lungs, and other internal organs continue to function without conscious thought. This is recognized by modern physiologists. The mechanism of movement in the form lies in the muscles and tendons. If the muscles are strong but the mind is not sharp, the movement will be slow despite great strength. If the muscles are strong and the mind is sharp, then it will be better. However, if suddenly faced with a strong opponent and need to act in haste, it is difficult to maintain composure. It requires a masterful technique. This is like a child who is just beginning to learn a craft. It is rare to have perfect coordination between the mind and the hands. However, for those who have practiced Xing Yi Quan for a long time, it is not difficult. Today's educators are doing their best to promote craftsmanship. The essence of craftsmanship lies in the coordination of mind and hand. Therefore, if one is skilled in the art of Xing Yi, it should be easier to learn a craft. From this point of view, the function of Xing Yi is limited to self-defense and fitness. However, there may be further benefits. If one concentrates Qi in the chest, breathing will not be difficult. If one concentrates Qi in the lower abdomen, one can maintain it for a long time without impeding breathing. Gradually accumulating Qi can make it more abundant, and it can be directed by the mind. When one strikes with a fist, one can guide the Qi to the fist. This is like using all the power in the body to focus on one point of the fist. The momentum is powerful and unstoppable. If one experiences discomfort, then one can guide the Qi to the affected area. The blood will flow, and the white blood cells can kill microorganisms and remove disease. The Qi is strong and fills the space between the two. One's spirits become more alert and confident. Is this not what Mencius said? Only in this way can one bear great responsibility for society and oneself without any regrets. This is just a brief summary. To truly understand it requires a perceptive mind.

Firstly, closing the mouth and touching the palate with the tongue causes saliva to be produced and swallowed, which helps to keep the qi from leaking out and prevents impurities in the air from entering the mouth. This should be done not only when practicing martial arts but also when not using the mouth. Touching the palate with the tongue produces saliva to prevent dryness in the mouth and throat.

Secondly, wrapping the elbow, lowering the shoulders, expanding the chest, and drumming the belly are essential techniques in Xingyi Quan. Wrapping the elbow causes the arm to bend slightly, allowing the force from the shoulder to be transmitted to the hand. This key point applies to all Xingyi Quan punches. For example, in the Pi Quan, the entire body's strength can only be delivered to the fingertips when this technique is applied. Those who believe that finger strength is weak must understand that the entire body's strength is concentrated in this technique. Without wrapping the elbow, the arm becomes stiff, and the force is limited to the arm, unable to be released outward. Beginners can test this themselves. Lowering the shoulders prevents Qi from floating and allows it to gather in the lower abdomen. Without lowering the shoulders, one cannot sustain for long. Drumming the belly gathers Qi in the lower abdomen. The human body has two main Qi storage areas, the lungs, and the lower abdomen below the navel. If Qi is stored in the lungs, it cannot be sustained for long and must be released through breathing. If Qi is stored in the lower abdomen, it will not interfere with breathing, as the lungs can continue to breathe without causing Qi to overflow. When practicing, one must expand the chest to ensure that the accumulated Qi does not obstruct breathing. For those who want to gather Qi in the lower abdomen and force the lung's Qi into the lower abdomen, they must suppress the chest to achieve this. This will result in undeveloped lungs and hindered breathing, which is harmful to the body. Therefore, even if Qi is gathered in the lower abdomen, the lungs must be allowed to expand naturally to avoid harm.

Thirdly, squeeze the legs together and grab the ground with the toes. Squeezing the legs together can prevent the body from tilting forward or backward. It is often seen that a strong man is defeated by a weaker but more agile opponent. Based on the strength of the strong man, he should be able to win the battle, but he often loses due to using force improperly. When he moves forward, he may lean his entire body forward without any support from behind, which allows the opponent to use his strength to defeat him. Grabbing the ground with the toes can make the body more stable.

In order for the eyes to be bright and agile and to be responsive to the hands and heart during a sparring match, it is essential to rely entirely on the action of the hands and heart, with the eyes being the most important. If the eyes are not bright and agile, they cannot respond to the hands and heart, and it is rare for a person to win. This is a well-known fact. However, how should the eyes be used during a sparring match? This is what needs to be studied.

1. When sparring, look up at the opponent's eyes. The direction of their eyes indicates the direction of their hands.
2. Look at the opponent's heart when they are at a medium distance. The movement of their hands will be in front of their heart.
3. Look down at the opponent's feet. The direction of their feet indicates their body's position.

1. The body is stable and the breath is even. When observing ordinary boxing practitioners, they often leap and kick with their legs, which is not without beauty and can be considered a form of exercise. However, it is not sufficient for sparring. Why is this so? Because I conserve my energy while endangering my opponent's safety. When two people spar, how can one spare a foot to kick when both feet are afraid of being unstable? If the kick misses, defeat is inevitable. Moreover, by calmly observing the opponent's movements with both eyes, one can respond accordingly. Why exhaust oneself by leaping and jumping? Such useless movements have no place in the form and intention of martial arts.

2. The boxing techniques are concise. In ordinary boxing, the movement of the arm is divided into a defensive move and an offensive move. If someone attacks me, I must defend first before attacking. But in the case of Xingyi, it is not like that. Attack is defense and defense is attack, one move for both. For example, let's examine the fist technique of the chopping punch. If someone attacks my heart with their left fist, regardless of the height of their punch, I just move forward to their right side, and use my right hand to chop as the splitting fist technique, blocking their arm. I have already defended myself. At the same time, as I move forward, my arm will brush past their arm at an angle and if their reaction is not quick enough, they will be hit by my punch. This is called "attack is defense". If their reaction is quick and they lift my punch, I will take advantage of their force to draw back my punch, gradually lowering it into a palm strike and then quickly turning it into a chopping punch, pushing forward their body. They will have no time to defend against it. This is because they will have to use a lot of force to lift my punch and they will not be able to retract their force in time. I will use their force to quickly attack them. I will make a circular motion and they will be hit by my punch. I attack them with one arm and they will not have time to defend themselves or attack me. This is not only defense but also offense. Isn't Xingyi Boxing really agile and convenient? Some may say that the crushing fist is very direct and may not have such a wonderful application. But the fact is that the crushing fist has two uses. If the opponent's punch is high, my punch

will come in from below, using an upward force to lift their arm. When my punch comes in at an angle, I will move forward to their side. Their punch will miss me and I can attack them with my punch. At the same time, I will not give up my forward strike. Then their punch will not have time to hit mine. Even if it does, they will not be able to hit it completely because I have already prepared for it. Their body will be hit by my punch. If the opponent's punch is low, my punch will come in from above, using a downward force to press down their arm. Their punch will be blocked and their arm will not be long enough to reach my body. My punch will brush past their punch and hit their body. Who says the crushing punch has only one use?

3. Strengthening the spirit through cultivating Qi can only be attained by those who practice internal exercises. Xing Yi emphasizes both internal and external exercises, as discussed in detail in Chapter 5.

In the summer of the fourth year of the Republic of China, I returned to the south and passed by the home of Yu Jie in my hometown. I read the Wumuquan manual that he had kept, which included nine essential principles and one section on sparring techniques. Although there were some mistakes in the wording, the writing was magnificent and truly the work of Wumu. The logic was profound and could only be understood by someone as accomplished as Wumu. I said, "This is an old Xingyi manual. With this divine inspiration, Xingyi martial arts will become more and more renowned as time goes on." I immediately copied it and brought it to the capital to share it with fellow martial arts enthusiasts from all over the world. Those who admire Wumu should cherish it and not lose it. Signed, Zheng Lianpu of Jiyuan School.

<u>**Chapter 1: Essentials 1**</u>

From ancient times, there must be unity in dispersement and harmony in division. Thus, the various things in the world each have their own affiliation, with countless strands and numerous sources. One thing may be dispersed into a myriad of variations, yet these variations all return to the one thing. There are necessities in all things, and the study of martial arts is also very complex. It involves a thousand variations and transformations, with no movement lacking in force, and no force lacking in energy. Although the forces may not be similar, they all return to the same energy. This energy extends from the top of the body to the soles of the feet, internally including the organs, tendons, and bones, and externally including the muscles, skin, and the hundreds of bones that make up the five senses. These are all interconnected, and even if broken, they will not come apart. When the upper body moves, the lower body follows, and when the lower body moves, the upper body leads. When both upper and lower move, the middle attacks, and when the middle moves, the upper and lower cooperate. The inside and outside are connected, and the front and back rely on each other. This is what is meant by unity. However, this cannot be forced, but must be achieved through sudden inspiration. One must be still and peaceful, like a mountain, but when the time comes to move, one must move like thunder or collapse, quickly and without hesitation. When still, one is completely still, with no sense of unevenness or disturbance in the upper and lower body. When moving, there is no dragging or hesitation, only a smooth and fluid motion, like water flowing downwards, unstoppable and unyielding, or like fire burning inside, sudden and unstoppable, without the need for thought or doubt. Indeed, it is a natural and effortless state that is difficult to attain. This comes from the accumulation of energy over time, and the diligent practice of skill. To truly understand the unity of the art, one must have a broad knowledge and strong intelligence, and reach a sudden realization without abandoning the effort to understand. There are no easy or difficult things in life, only the effort that we put into them. We cannot rush, nor can we wait. We must take each step carefully, and advance one by one. Only then will the joints and bones of the body have a smooth connection, and the inside and outside will be linked as one. In the end, all the bones and organs of the body will return to one energy, with unity in dispersement and harmony in division.

There are those who discuss the practice of punching in the world, and also discuss Qi. Qi is the master of unity, but it can be divided into two parts, which are known as breathing. Breathing is Yin and Yang. Punching cannot be without movement and stillness, and Qi cannot be without breathing. Inhaling is Yin, and exhaling is Yang. The main Yin is stillness, and the main Yang is movement. Rising is Yang, and descending is Yin. Yang Qi rises and becomes Yang, and Yang Qi descends and becomes Yin. Yin Qi descends and becomes Yin, and Yin Qi rises and becomes Yang. This is the division of Yin and Yang. What is clear and turbid is that rising is clear, and descending is turbid. Clear Qi rises, and turbid Qi descends. Clear is Yang, and turbid is Yin. To nourish Yin with Yang is to unify Qi. Speaking generally, it is all Qi, but speaking specifically, it is Yin and Yang. Qi cannot be without Yin and Yang, just as people cannot be without movement and stillness, the nose cannot be without breathing, and the mouth cannot be without intake and outflow. This is the principle of treating and circulating without difficulty. Therefore, Qi is divided into two parts, but it actually exists as one. Those who aspire to this path should not be constrained by this.

# Chapter 3: Essentials 3

The breath is essential to the body, and cannot be separated into two. Breathing is the same as Yin and Yang, with inhalation being Yin and exhalation being Yang. Yin is associated with stillness, while Yang is associated with movement. Upward movement is Yang, while downward movement is Yin. If the breath is clear, it rises upwards; if it is turbid, it descends. Clear breath is Yang, while turbid breath is Yin. Yin nourishes Yang, and they are all part of Qi. Qi cannot exist without Yin and Yang, just as the body cannot exist without stillness and movement, breathing, and circulation.

The body is divided into three sections: upper, middle, and lower. The head is the upper section, the body is the middle section, and the legs are the lower section. The upper section can be divided into three subsections: the upper section is the Heavenly Palace, the middle section is the nose, and the lower section is the sea of Qi. The middle section can be divided into three subsections: the upper section is the chest, the middle section is the abdomen, and the lower section is the Dan Tian. The lower section can be divided into three subsections: the tip of the foot, the middle section is the knee, and the root of the thigh is the root section.

The arms are also divided into three sections: the tip of the hand, the middle section is the elbow, and the root section is the shoulder. Similarly, the fingers are the tip of the hand, the palm is the middle section, and the root section is the wrist. All of these sections are important, and ignoring any of them can lead to negative consequences.

When it comes to the movement of Qi, the tip of the limbs should move first, followed by the middle section, and the root section should follow. Although each section is important, the body should be seen as a whole, with all four limbs and 100 bones forming a unified structure. Therefore, the division of the body into upper, middle, and lower sections is arbitrary and should not be taken too seriously.

**<u>Chapter 4: Essentials 4</u>**

Apart from discussing the body and energy, let's move on to the topic of "shao" (i.e. the extremities). "Shao" refers to the residual threads of the body, which are not initially discussed when talking about the body or energy. The use of energy is not limited to the body; if it is, it will be empty and ineffective. If it does not take shape in the extremities, it will be both real and empty. It is necessary to discuss the extremities, but this only touches upon the extremities of the body, not yet on the extremities of the energy. What are the four extremities? They are where energy is released. Although they are not classified in the Five Elements or related to the four limbs, it seems unnecessary to discuss them. However, the extremity of blood is related to energy. Although we do not need to discuss energy based on blood, we cannot separate energy from blood. Without blood, we cannot reach the extremities. The tip of the tongue is the extremity of the flesh, and the flesh is the bag of energy. If energy cannot take shape in the extremities of the flesh, it cannot be fully contained in the body. Therefore, we must try to clench our teeth with our tongue to make the extremity of the flesh sufficient. As for the extremity of the bone, it is the teeth, and the extremity of the tendon is the fingernail. Energy is generated in the bones and linked to the tendons. If it is not related to the teeth, it is not related to the extremities of the tendons either. If we want our hands to be sufficient, we need to strengthen our teeth and fingernails. If we can do this, then the four extremities are sufficient, and the energy is also sufficient. How can there be emptiness and reality, reality and emptiness?

In martial arts, the power of striking is based on the concept of qi, which stems from the five organs that form the shape of a human body. The five organs, namely the heart, liver, spleen, lungs, and kidneys, are the source of life and energy, each with their unique characteristics represented by fire, wood, earth, metal, and water, respectively. The position of the lungs channel is at the chest and is considered the covering of all other organs. When the lungs channel moves, the other organs cannot remain still. The heart is located in the middle of the chest and is protected by the lungs. The liver and spleen are located on the left and right sides between the ribs, respectively, while the kidneys are located at the back, along the spine. The waist is where the two kidneys are positioned, and it is the root of all organs, especially for the five organs. The internal organs have their specific locations while other body parts, such as the top of the head, the back, and the neck, also have their specific corresponding organs. The forehead, for instance, corresponds to the stomach meridian, and the two eyes correspond to the liver, with the upper part of the eyes belonging to the spleen and the lower part to the stomach. The white part of the eye corresponds to the lungs, while the black part corresponds to the liver. The nose corresponds to the central earth and is the source of all living things, especially the main point for the Qi. The human body's vital energy and blood converge in the central point between the eyebrows, which is called the Yintang acupoint. The lips are related to the Chongmai meridian, which runs from the pubic area to the mouth, and the space under the lips is the Renmai meridian. The neck connects all the channels and collaterals of the five organs, providing a passage for the Qi to circulate and nourish the body. The shoulders correspond to the lungs, the elbows to the kidneys, and the limbs to the spleen.

The heart and mind unite, the mind and Qi unite, the Qi and strength unite; these are the internal three unions. The hands and feet unite, the elbows and knees unite, the shoulders and hips unite; these are the external three unions. Together they form the six unions. The left hand and right foot unite, the left elbow and right knee unite, the left shoulder and right hip unite, and vice versa. The head and hands unite, the hands and body unite, the body and steps unite; these are not external unions. The heart and eyes unite, the liver and tendons unite, the spleen and flesh unite, the lungs and body unite, the kidneys and bones unite; these are not internal unions. It's not just about the six unions, but also the five forms and hundred bones, which are all used in this. In summary, one movement without movement, one union without disunity; using all the parts of the body.

The head is the leader of the six yangs and the master of the whole body. All five senses and hundred bones rely on it. Therefore, the head cannot be neglected. The hands are the leaders and have their foundation in the shoulders. If the shoulders do not advance, then the hands will retreat and not move forward. This is why the shoulders are important to advance. The Qi gathers at the wrists and the joints are at the waist. If the waist does not advance, then the Qi will become weak and not solid. This is why the waist is important to advance. The intention penetrates the whole body and the movement is in the steps. If the steps do not advance, then the intention will be useless. This is why the steps must advance. Also, the left must advance to the right, and the right must advance to the left. These are the seven advances, and this is the area where one must concentrate their efforts. If the advance is not reached, the whole body will not be coordinated and will lack a unified movement.

What is the method of body movement? It is only vertical, horizontal, high, and low, forward, backward, and reverse. When moving vertically, expand your momentum and move forward without turning back. When moving horizontally, wrap your strength and open up without hindrance. When moving high, elevate your body and make it appear taller. When moving low, lower your body and make it appear compressed. When you should advance, exhaust your body and boldly charge forward. When you should retreat, lead your energy and turn around to assume a crouching position. When reversing, look back to the rear; the rear is now the front. When looking to the sides, make the sides afraid to confront you. But do not be constrained by these methods. You must first assess the opponent's strength and weaknesses, and manipulate your own mechanisms accordingly. There are times to move vertically and times to move horizontally, as movements vary with the situation and cannot be treated the same. There are times to move high and times to move low, as height and depth change with the situation and cannot be held to a fixed standard. At times you should advance, and not retreat and squander your energy; at times you should retreat, and encourage your advance. Even when reversing and looking back, make the back appear as the front, and when looking to the sides, make the sides appear as not worth confronting. In short, the mechanism is in the eyes, the flexibility is in the mind, and the crucial point is to grasp the essence, so that when you move forward, all four limbs move naturally, and when you move backward, all one hundred bones remain immobile. The method of body movement can be left aside and not discussed.

The human body's five organs and hundred bones are responsible for movement, but it is footwork that makes it possible. Footwork is the basis for all bodily movements and the pivot point for movements. Thus, in a combat situation, the body's origin is in the footwork, which is its pillar. While the hands can adapt to changes, the footwork serves as the turning point for hands. Without footwork, it is impossible to create the momentum needed for attack and defense or show the subtleties of change. The eyes hold the mechanism, and the changes come from the mind. To make various movements without being trapped, the commander is none other than the footwork. However, it should not be forced, and movements should come from an empty mind while excitement comes from being unaware. When the body desires movement, footwork assists it in circling. When the hands move, footwork urges them to move quickly, and the body and footwork move in unison.

Footwork can be divided into front and back, each with its own position. Stepping forward with the front foot and following with the back foot creates a position. However, if the front foot becomes the back foot, and vice versa, there is no natural position. When discussing the potential of a fist, footwork is the key factor, determining its agility. The effectiveness of footwork is immense. The fist is called "Xin Yi" (mind and intention), where intention arises from the mind, and the fist follows the intention. It is essential to understand oneself and others and adapt to changes as they come. Once the mind and energy unite, the limbs move in unison.

When attacking, the fist should not be more than five feet away or less than three feet away. The goal is to hit the opponent, taking one step and one punch, regardless of front, back, left, or right. The subtlety lies in making the punch invisible, fast as an arrow, and sounding like thunder. In close combat, swift and decisive action is crucial. One should move like an arrow, strike like the wind, and use grappling techniques if necessary. Your movements should be fluid and unpredictable, like lightning, and guard both sides to avoid being caught off guard. Strike high and low, aiming for the opponent's center. Be swift like a tiger and quick like a hawk, move like the waves and overturn like a storm.

In martial arts, skill determines the battle's outcome. Therefore, every step should be measured carefully, and every strike should be executed with precision. To move forward, use your right leg and step forward with your left foot. When approaching your opponent, your body and hands should move together in unison. To win, all four extremities must coordinate, and if you can't win, you must retreat and try again. With strategy and skill, a thunderbolt moves with great speed, and a wise fighter clarifies their intentions to use a crisis to their advantage.

# Chapter 10: Fighting Techniques

Take right and advance left, take left and advance right. When stepping forward, the foot should first touch the ground at the root, with the toes grabbing the ground. The step should be stable, the body should be solemn. When punching, it should be heavy and powerful. When withdrawing the hand, it should become a fist, which should be tightly coiled. When using a hold, it should have Qi. The breath should be even, and the mind should control the in and out movements. The eyes, hands, and feet should follow the mind, neither too greedy nor too restrained, the elbow should fall into the elbow socket, and the hand should fall into the hand socket. The right foot should be the first to move forward, the arm pointing forward, this is called changing step.

Punch from the heart, use body force to drive the hand, use the hand to control the heart. Advance with each step, strike with each punch, and one movement will follow the other. With precision and force, grip everything tightly as if grasping a cannon, with great power. Whether it's lifting, pressing, swinging, cutting, charging, striking, elbowing, shoulder hitting, hip hitting, head hitting, advancing, retreating, following, or turning, every strike should follow one breath. Strike first at the centerline, this is called skill. The joints should be aligned, otherwise there will be no strength. The hand should be agile, or it will change unpredictably. Punch quickly, or it will be delayed. Raise the hand flexibly, or it will be slow.

Follow the opponent closely, or it will be ineffective. Have a poisonous intention, or it will not be accurate. Move the hands and feet nimbly, or there will be danger. Be precise in intention, or be foolish. When making a move, be fierce like an eagle and have a courageous heart. The outer appearance should be brave. Mastery requires practice, do not fear doubts and uncertainties. Be brave in mind and cautious in appearance. Be calm like a scholar but explosive like thunder. Observe the opponent's movements carefully, and respond accordingly.

Kicks to the head, punches to the body, narrow stances and explosive movements are all essential. Switching steps diagonally, intercepting and reversing the opponent, kicking and stretching legs, and watching out for attacks from unexpected directions are also important. Attacks must be both fast and accurate. Timing and footwork must be coordinated. A slow hand is the same as no hand. Timing is critical, and movements must be coordinated.

Fakes and feints are important tactics. Use elbows and knees for close range, and kicks for longer distances.

Observe the opponent's movements and respond appropriately. Coordinating hands and feet is crucial for victory. Striking people must be exquisite, with hands and feet arriving together. Striking people is like uprooting grass; striking above targets the throat, striking below targets the groin. The left and right ribs are at the center. Striking from a distance of three meters is not considered far; when close, it is only within one inch. When the body moves, it should be like a collapsing wall; when the feet land, it should be like a tree taking root. The hands should rise straight up like a cannon firing, and the body should move like a live snake. When striking the head, the tail should respond; when striking the tail, the head should respond. Striking the joints will cause both ends to respond. When striking forward, one should also consider guarding the rear. Knowing how to advance requires also knowing how to retreat. The mind should be as quick as a horse, and the kidneys should move as fast as the wind.

During practice, it should feel as if there is someone in front; during sparring, it should feel as if there is no one there. The front hand should be raised, and the rear hand should be urged tightly. The front foot should be lifted, and the rear foot should follow closely. When facing hands, don't see hands; when facing elbows, don't see elbows. If you see emptiness, don't strike; if you see emptiness, don't go up. The fist should not strike emptiness when rising, nor should it strike emptiness when falling. When the hand rises, the foot should land; when the foot lands, the hand should rise.

The mind should take precedence, the intent should win over the opponent, the body should attack the opponent, and the steps should surpass the opponent. The front leg should resemble a kneeling position, and the rear leg should resemble a standstill. The head should be raised, the chest should be shown, the waist should be extended, and the dantian should move the Qi. From head to toe, there should be one continuous flow of Qi. If one is frightened and nervous, one cannot win. If one cannot observe words and expressions, one cannot guard against the opponent. If one cannot move first, one is the student; if one moves last, one is the younger student. Encourage oneself to move forward, and do not allow oneself to retreat. The three joints should stop, the three points should be illuminated, and the four tips should be level.

Understanding the three hearts requires more power, understanding the three joints requires more direction, understanding the four tips requires more precision, and understanding the five elements requires more Qi. Understanding the three joints without greed or lack, the rise and fall, advance and retreat should be diverse. Three repetitions and nine turns make up one movement. One must be governed by a single mind, related to the five elements, and moved by two Qi. Practice constantly, and do not neglect it day or night. When practicing, strive diligently; after long practice, it will become natural. These are sincere words, not empty talk.

According to the Yan Ji Xing Yi, it was passed down from Shan You, and the Shan You Xing Yi was passed down from Zhongzhou. Therefore, the scattered Xing Yi Quan scriptures seen throughout north and south of the Yellow River are also a result of circumstances. However, due to the passage of time and the vast distance, there is no unified system, and there are many errors in the transmission of the written word. The ten volumes of the original family are not enough to fully illustrate the entirety of Xing Yi martial arts. Nevertheless, this article is a valuable treasure with its limited scope. Although I am not talented, I dare to take this as a congratulation for my own path.

-    Shu Lu, Li Jianqiu.

www.ingramcontent.com/pod-product-compliance
Lightning Source LLC
Chambersburg PA
CBHW051826250726
48659CB00005B/1692